T0093031

Phytocosmetics and Cosmetic Science

CRC FOCUS

Phytocosmetics and Cosmetic Science

Edited by Nattaya Lourith, PhD

Phytocosmetics and Cosmeceuticals Research Group
School of Cosmetic Science, Mae Fah Luang University
Chiang Rai, Thailand

Karl W.K. Tsim, PhD

Shenzhen Key Laboratory of Edible and Medicinal Bioresources
HKUST Shenzhen Research Institute
Shenzen, China

and

Division of Life Science and Center for Chinese Medicine
The Hong Kong University of Science and Technology
Hong Kong, China

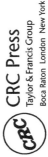 CRC Press
Taylor & Francis Group
Boca Raton London New York

CRC Press is an imprint of the
Taylor & Francis Group, an **informa** business

First edition published 2021
by CRC Press
6000 Broken Sound Parkway NW, Suite 300, Boca Raton, FL 33487-2742

and by Taylor & Francis Group
2 Park Square, Milton Park, Abingdon, Oxon, OX14 4RN

© 2021 Taylor & Francis Group, LLC

CRC Press is an imprint of Taylor & Francis Group, LLC

Library of Congress Cataloging-in-Publication Data

Names: Lourith, Nattaya, editor. | Tsim, Karl Wah-Keung, editor.
Title: Phytocosmetics and cosmetic science / edited by Nattaya Lourith, Karl W.K. Tsim.
Description: First edition. | Boca Raton : CRC Press, 2021. | Includes bibliographical references and index. | Summary: "This guide acts as a concise and quick reference from key researchers and an up-to-date guide to translation into practice, providing an easy-to-consult resource on a topic of great current interest"— Provided by publisher.
Identifiers: LCCN 2021011698 (print) | LCCN 2021011699 (ebook) | ISBN 9780367619763 (hardback) | ISBN 9780367619930 (paperback) | ISBN 9781003107385 (ebook)
Subjects: MESH: Phytochemicals | Cosmetics | Plants, Medicinal
Classification: LCC RS160 (print) | LCC RS160 (ebook) | NLM QV 766 | DDC 615.3/21—dc23
LC record available at https://lccn.loc.gov/2021011698
LC ebook record available at https://lccn.loc.gov/2021011699

ISBN: 978-0-367-61976-3 (hbk)
ISBN: 978-0-367-61993-0 (pbk)
ISBN: 978-1-003-10738-5 (ebk)

Typeset in Times
by KnowledgeWorks Global Ltd.

Contents

Preface

Cosmetics have been used for cleanliness and aesthetic proposes that boost individuals' self-esteem and confidence. They have been therefore involved in our lives from ancient times, and the preferences between and expectations of cosmetics are continually in flux with advances in technology and revolutions in the scientific basis. There are many different disciplines that contribute to the success of cosmetics from the laboratory until they reach consumers. With regard to our current society and the probable future, natural products are much in focus, including those for cosmetics, and in particular, phytocosmetics – cosmetic preparations in any dosage form, composed of plants or plant extracts (as a total extract or in crude form), and selected active principles or isolated pure compounds from plants.

This text looks at the application of plant-derived ingredients in cosmetics by their functional and active tasks. With up-to-date and comprehensive content, the chapters have been written by authors who play an important role in cosmetic science. We would like to express our deepest gratitude to the contributors who kindly share their knowledge and interests in this book. We wish to thank our publisher, CRC Press, Robert Peden, and his colleagues for all the suggestions and support they have given.

Nattaya Lourith
Karl W.K. Tsim

Contributors

Aviva S.F. Chow
Department of Pharmacology and
Pharmacy
Li Ka Shing Faculty School of
Medicine
The University of Hong Kong
Hong Kong, China

Geoffrey A. Cordell
Natural Products Inc.
Evanston, Illinois
and
Department of Pharmaceutics
College of Pharmacy
University of Florida
Gainesville, Florida

Sharna-kay Daley
Natural Products Inc.
Evanston, Illinois

Maggie S.S. Guo
Shenzhen Key Laboratory of Edible
and Medicinal Bioresources
HKUST Shenzhen Research Institute
Shenzhen, China
Division of Life Science and Center
for Chinese Medicine
The Hong Kong University of
Science and Technology
Hong Kong, China

Mayuree Kanlayavattanakul
Phytocosmetics and Cosmeceuticals
Research Group
School of Cosmetic Science
Mae Fah Luang University
Chiang Rai, Thailand

Yushi Katsuyama
CIEL Co. Ltd.
Sagamihara-shi, Kanagawa
Tokyo University of Technology
Hachioji-shi, Tokyo, Japan

Queenie W.S. Lai
Shenzhen Key Laboratory of Edible
and Medicinal Bioresources
HKUST Shenzhen Research Institute
Shenzhen, China
Division of Life Science and Center
for Chinese Medicine
The Hong Kong University of
Science and Technology
Hong Kong, China

Nattaya Lourith, PhD
Phytocosmetics and Cosmeceuticals
Research Group
School of Cosmetic Science, Mae
Fah Luang University
Chiang Rai, Thailand

Hitoshi Masaki
CIEL Co. Ltd. Sagamihara-shi,
    Kanagawa,
Tokyo University of Technology
Tokyo, Japan

Henry H. Y. Tong
School of Health Sciences and
    Sports
Macao Polytechnic Institute
Macao, China

Karl W.K. Tsim
Shenzhen Key Laboratory of Edible
    and Medicinal Bioresources
HKUST Shenzhen Research Institute
Shenzen, China
Division of Life Science Center for
    Chinese Medicine
The Hong Kong University of
    Science and Technology
Hong Kong, China

M. Pilar Vinardell
Department of Biochemistry and
    Physiology
Faculty of Pharmacy
Universitat de Barcelona
Barcelona, Spain

Qiyun Wu
Shenzhen Key Laboratory of Edible
    and Medicinal Bioresources
HKUST Shenzhen Research Institute
Shenzhen, China
Division of Life Science and Center
    for Chinese Medicine
The Hong Kong University of
    Science and Technology
Hong Kong, China

1

Introduction to Cosmetic Science and Phytocosmetics

Nattaya Lourith and Mayuree Kanlayavattanakul

Contents

1.1 COSMETIC SCIENCE

1.1.1 Introduction and Definitions

Cosmetics are the products applied to the human body (i.e. skin, hair, and nails) to promote cleanliness and aesthetic aspects/beauty, with an association with attractiveness or altering the appearance without affecting structure or function. Cosmetics are therefore different from drugs used for healing, curing, or prevention of disease. Although the physical appearance or dosage form of cosmetics and drug are similar, those of cosmetics must meet the users' preference or perception as regards odor, color, and texture. Accordingly, the cognitive process about cosmetics' characteristics, which delineates the symbolic value or positive emotional feeling, is of importance as well. Sensory assessment of cosmetics is therefore one of the hallmarks of the efficient product, which is perceptible by the users. Thus, multidisciplinary fields converge for a successful cosmetic product with a development process starting from the laboratory, through production, until it is available for the consumers. Science combines with law, regulation, and business management to integrate fruitfully in the cosmetics industry.

Cosmetics are usually noted to be the same sort of product as drugs in the sense of the consumers' awareness. Nonetheless, cosmetic regulation varies greatly internationally [1–4], as illustrated in Figure 1.1A. Some can be regarded as cosmetic or over-the-counter (OTC) products, others as quasi-drugs or special purpose cosmetics, others as drugs, depending on the law and regulation of the country, state, or union. It should be noted that some products can be classified as either cosmetics or not cosmetics; the quantity of an ingredient distinguishes if that product is classified as a cosmetic or not. Some ingredients are for medicinal uses; others could be supplied for both drugs and cosmetics. In the latter case, if some of the ingredient has been incorporated into the preparation at a concentration that makes it incapable of a medicinal or therapeutic effect, it is accounted as a cosmetics. However, in some cases, additional concern about the origin/nature of an ingredient causes different categorization. In addition, some regulations take into account the method of product application, dosage form, and appearance. Thus, cosmetic formulators are strongly recommended to consult the exact regulations for where the product is planned to be marketed.

Successful cosmetics depend on various branches of science. Cosmetic science integrates knowledge from chemistry, biology, physics, physiology, psychology, and computer science. Chemistry plays an important role in cosmetic

(A)

Cosmetic Classification				
ASEAN	Drug	Cosmetics		
China	Drug	Non-special purpose cosmetics		Special purpose cosmetics
EU	Drug	Cosmetics		
Japan	Drug	Quasi-Drug	Medicated Cosmetics	Cosmetics
USA	Drug	OTC	Cosmetics	

Product	ASEAN	China	EU	Japan	USA
Anti-perspirant	Cosmetics	Special purpose cosmetics	Cosmetics	Quasi-Drug	OTC
Anti-acne	Drug	Special purpose cosmetics	Drug	Quasi-Drug	OTC
Anti-dandruff	Drug	Special purpose cosmetics	Cosmetics	Quasi-Drug	Drug/Cosmetics
Hair dye	Cosmetics	Special purpose cosmetics	Cosmetics	Cosmetics	Cosmetics
Moisturizer	Cosmetics	Non-special purpose cosmetics	Cosmetics	Cosmetics	Cosmetics
Mouthwash	Cosmetics	Special purpose cosmetics	Cosmetics	Quasi-Drug	Drug/Cosmetics
Sunscreen	Cosmetics	Special purpose cosmetics	Cosmetics	Cosmetics	OTC

(B)

(C)

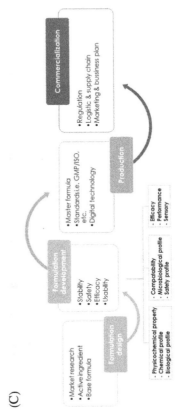

FIGURE 1.1 (A) Classification of cosmetics, (B) Quality parameters and dosage forms, and (C) Cosmetic development flow.

ingredients in the aspects of preparation and quality of the ingredient. Of these, quality refers to safety, stability, usability, and efficacy (Figure 1.1B). Accordingly, organic chemistry, inorganic chemistry, analytical chemistry, physical chemistry, biochemistry, and polymer chemistry are all applied in cosmetics (Figure 1.1C). That is the reason why cosmetic science used to be categorized as formulation chemistry, a subset of applied chemistry. In fact, creating a product fits with the users' preference and demand does not straightforwardly rely on formulation. Development of the cosmetic product suitable for the body site to be used, frequency of use, and the users' feeling are also key aspects in cosmetics development. Thus, physiology and psychology are the most concerning issues for cosmetics in the point of sensory evaluation, and statistics is clearly fundamental for these fields. Furthermore, computer science is one of the important fields in cosmetics for laboratory and manufacturing scales production, including for packaging and labeling designs as well as for marketing communications and commercial advertisements. Taking into account its multidisciplinary fields, "cosmetic science" is a uniquely successful integration of sciences and arts.

1.1.2 Cosmetic Dosage Form

Cosmetics can be presented in a variety of formulations that can be simply categorized by the body area for application [5, 6]. Cosmetics for facial, skin, hair, and nail care, including fragrance and makeup products, are therefore common. These can be used for cleansing, conditioning, hydrating, moisturizing, nourishing, odor masking, perfuming, and decorating (these different types of formulation can be marked with commercial buzzwords). Cosmetics are best grouped on the basis of their physicochemical properties or dosage form i.e. liquid or solution, semi-solid, and solid (Figure 1.1B).

Cosmetic liquids or solutions are those that are a clear, non-viscous liquid. Astringent, essence, perfume, makeup remover, mouthwash, tonic, and toner are examples of cosmetics in the dosage form of liquid or solution. Semi-solid cosmetics are those dispersing systems that are liquids dispersed in liquids or solids dispersed in liquids or liquids dispersed in solid. These systems are called emulsion, gel, and suspension, respectively. The dispersal is either two-phase (oil in water, o/w; water in oil, w/o; silicone in water, si/w; water in silicone, w/si) or multiphase (e.g. o/w/o, w/o/w/o, etc.). The dosage form of semi-solid is the major form of cosmetic formulations – for example, cream, lotion, serum, shampoo, concealer, foundation, and nail lacquer. Solid cosmetics include powder (loose and compressed), brusher, lipstick, antiperspirant, deodorant, bath-bomb, scrub, mud, clay, etc.

Different cosmetic dosage forms differ not only in appearance but also in physicochemical property, frequency, concentration and duration of use, and exposure type. This will be specified by the ingredients and microbial specification of the preparation as well.

1.1.3 Cosmetic Quality Overview

In the course of cosmetic business, there are several steps and issues, which are multidisciplinary related and needed to be addressed to ensure cosmetics' quality, especially during the course of formulation development [5–7]. The formulation must be evaluated in several parameters (as depicted in Figure 1.1C) for quality assurance throughout the cosmetic product life cycle. The evaluation protocols are delineated by the international guidelines (i.e. GMP, ISO, IEC, ASTM, ANSI, BS, EN), which are described in detail in accordance with the product.

1.2 PHYTOCOSMETICS

Herbal products have long been used in several applications both for beneficial aspects in terms of food and medicinal herbs and for contrary uses as poisonous herbs. The common and well-known herbs used for food are garlic, lemon, peppermint, and ginger. The medicinal applications of aloe, ginkgo, and ginseng are well-recognized for their pharmacotherapeutic effects, while some mushrooms are toxic to humans. Of all the herbal products known for therapeutic effects, plants are the most used.

It is well-documented that there are positive effects for human health from plant-derived products in Ayurvedic, Chinese, Indusynunic, Islamic or Unani-Tibb, Kampo, and Oriental recipes originating in India, China, Pakistan, Middle East, Japan, and Korea and other Asian countries. In addition, the traditional medicines in European and African countries relied on plants that are also now incorporated in Herbalism or Homeopathy. "Plant" – in the Latin from, "phyto", – is therefore included in several words, for example phytochemistry (the chemistry of plants, plant processes, and plant products), or phytoremediation (the treatment of pollutants or waste with plant or phytotherapy) or phytoremedies (health remedy or disease treatment with plant).

Plants are popular for health promotion, and similarly most applications of plants in cosmetics are popular world-wide and recognized in the term of "phytocosmetics." Phytocosmetics therefore refers to a cosmetics preparation in any dosage form comprising a plant (i.e. plant extract – total extract or crude), selected active principles, or isolated pure compounds from plants. Plant-derived ingredients in cosmetics are applied according to their functional or active tasks. A functional task is defined by their function in the formulation technology, such as film-former, gelling agent, thickener, suspending agent, conditioner, and emulsifier; this mainly relies on their physicochemical properties. Phytocosmetics with an active task are those with a positive effect on the aesthetic conditions of skin and hair, i.e. anti-aging, skin lightening, skin hydrating/moisturizing, anti-greasiness, anti-dandruff, anti-microbial, hair color covering, anti-hair loss, and so forth. Consumer awareness, acceptance, and demand for natural cosmetics are therefore clearly helpful for phytocosmetics. The expectations for phytocosmetics in the market are dramatically increasing each year in regard to their perceived safety and efficacy, joined with the consumers' desire for eco-friendly and sustainable products. Much work is therefore undertaken in academic research societies, research institutes and industrial sectors, in search of new discoveries to help progress in technology and development, which in turn helps increase demand.

1.2.1   General Information Requirements for Phytocosmetics

In order to develop safe and efficient phytocosmetics, it is necessary to have information to ensure quality – both basic data requirements and consumer awareness.

1.2.2   Basic Data Requirements

1. *Plant property and activity*

In the search for a candidate plant to be used as a phytocosmetics, the first step would be to conduct a literature review to determine if that plant has been traditionally documented in any remedies with cutaneous and aesthetic applications. The botanical identity can confirm and widen such literature searches. Some plants used in different cultures have had their properties recorded – for example, they may regulate sebum, be anti-bacterial, anti-inflammatory/anti-irritant, soothing/calming, skin healing and regeneration, stimulate skin regeneration, stimulate collagen production or inhibit breakdown, protect against UV and harsh conditions, be anti-oxidant/free radical scavenger, phytopheromones, moisturizing/nourishing/smoothing, circulatory stimulant, anti-swelling, astringent, etc. Searches should also be made for analytical data and claims substantiation (i.e. chemical measurement on actives and contaminants, *in vitro*, *ex vivo* or cellular, and *in vivo* data). Finally, the exact plant part to use and preparation of the plant's extract are points of great importance to ensure its phytocosmetic potency.

2. *Safety*

Several plants and plant extracts may be shown in a search for their function and activities on the basis of their biologically active components and *in vitro* and cellular properties. Nevertheless, if the plant lacks toxicological information, the plant or its extract will be disqualified for use. Although the toxicological information for a cosmetic ingredient is not as strict as those for a medicinal product, this sort of information is still necessary. Toxicological information includes skin and eye irritation and sensitization, as well as the possible contaminants i.e. pesticides, herbicides, heavy metals, and impurities. Furthermore, there may be a possible interaction with another cosmetic ingredient available. In addition, microbiological specification of the plant and/or plant extract is needed to ensure its safety, and if it may be an allergen.

3. *Formulation*

To formulate phytocosmetics, the physicochemical properties of the ingredient – pH, miscibility, color – are vital, for compatibility of the ingredient with the available cosmetic raw materials. In addition, the ingredient itself has to show stability, which can be assessed by several conditions (i.e. an accelerated stability test including freeze-thaw [−20°C and +25°C] cycles and high-low temperatures [45°C and 4°C] storage). In addition, there should be long-term stability following storage (e.g. 60–90 days at 45°C or 4°C, 5–6 months at 37°C and 12–18 months under ambient condition or under specific recommended storage condition). Consistency is also necessary in certain quality parameters (i.e. physicochemical property, phytocosmetic active, biological activity, and safety referring stability of the phytocosmetics).

1.2.3 Consumer Awareness

The success of a phytocosmetics is not only determined by its activity, efficacy and safety; consumer's awareness is also a vital issue. Consumers are currently interested in many aspects of their consumable products, including those for personal care, and phytocosmetics need to rely not only on being animal friendly products, GMO-free certificates, and environmental responsibility, but also sustainability and social responsibility. Adaptive marketing communication of cosmetics and phytocosmetics should therefore directly rely on consumer's awareness and expand to fit with the consumers' beliefs about plants in different parts of the world, whether documented in traditional herbal medicine and those from specific geographical sources and/or extreme environments. The end-result can be extraordinarily powerful.

1.3 CONCLUSION

In this book, the term phytocosmetics refers to a phytocosmetic active ingredient and a cosmetic formulation containing the phytocosmetic active. Chapters cover the ethnopharmacological sources of plants to be explored for phytocosmetic uses, especially traditional Chinese medicine, as well as the phytocosmetic actives for skin, hair, and malodorant applications. Assessment of safety and efficiency of phytocosmetics is also covered. Furthermore, the important issue of delivery technology and safety are addressed. Possible future developments of social and consumer awareness on sustainable issues are also summarized.

REFERENCES

1. CFDA. Regulation of cosmetics. http://samr.cfda.gov.cn/WS01/CL1028/
2. CFDA. Detection method for prohibited substances in cosmetics. http://samr.cfda.gov.cn/WS01/CL1192/
3. EU. Cosmetic legislation. https://ec.europa.eu/growth/sectors/cosmetics/legislation_en
4. USFDA. Code of Federal Regulations Sections for Cosmetics Labeling (CFR Title 21). https://www.ecfr.gov/cgi-bin/text-idx?SID=be3da3168a6d8dc1164616a51e3ee872&mc=true&tpl=/ecfrbrowse/Title21/21cfrv7_02.tpl#0
5. Barel AO, Paye M, Maibach HI. Handbook of cosmetic science and technology. 4th edition. Florida: CRC Press, 2014.
6. Mitsui T. New cosmetic science. Tokyo: Elsevier, 1997.
7. SCCS. The SCCS's notes of guidance for the testing of cosmetic substances and their safety evaluation. 8th revision. 2012.

2

Phytocosmetics Derived from Traditional Chinese Medicine

Qiyun Wu, Queenie W.S. Lai, Maggie S.S. Guo, and Karl W.K. Tsim

Contents

2.1 THE ORIGIN OF TRADITIONAL CHINESE MEDICINE IN COSMETOLOGY

Traditional Chinese Medicine (TCM) is said to be based on "Huangdi Neijing" (475–221 BC) [1] and "Bencao Gangmu" (1594 AD), two of the historical books describing its theory and usage. The principle of TCM is considering the holistic interaction of the human body and external surroundings as a whole: this close interaction promotes body health through a balance of "Yin" and "Yang," the two opposing forces, as suggested in Taoism. The imbalance of the two forces in the human leads to illness, including skin problems. TCM could then be used to restore the harmony by removing the intrinsic and/or extrinsic causes.

The development of TCM in cosmetology can be generally divided into four historical periods of dynasties in China: (i) antiquity to pre-Qin dynasty (221–206 BC); (ii) Qin/Han dynasties and Three Kingdom period (189–263 AD); (iii) Wei, Jin, Northern and Southern dynasties to Tang dynasties (581–907 AD); and (iv) Song to Qing dynasty (1644–1912 AD) [2]. In the ancient period, the primary application of TCM in skin mainly focused on curing skin diseases, maintaining youthfulness of skin, and promoting facial attractiveness. Ancient cosmetics in China were tailored for makeup, skincare, nail polish, hair nourishment, and body fragrance: besides, the Chinese applied different colors and scents, derived from TCM, onto their body to represent their social classes [3]. TCM in cosmetology presumably began before the pre-Qin dynasty (before 221 BC), where the theoretical concepts and relationships among meridian, "Zang-Fu" and "Qi-Blood," as well as the relationship with facial appearance, had been recorded. In line to this notion, the etiology and pathogenesis of skin diseases had been described in ancient literatures, e.g. "Classic of Mountains and Seas" (400 BC), "Huangdi Neijing" (475–221 BC), "Nan Jing" (25–220 AD)." These texts summarized the medicinal experience of ancient Chinese in skin treatment.

2.2 THE PRINCIPLE OF TCM IN DERMATOLOGY

The theory of TCM has a distinctive explanation for dermatological diseases and problems. The following examples from Chinese medicinal literatures indicate the knowledge of the ancient Chinese in treating skin diseases. Acne vulgaris is a common skin disorder in the form of pimples or blackheads on face.

In the book chapter of "*Suwen*" of "*Huangdi Neijing*," the acne symptom was proposed to be controlled by the "*Lung*" channel, and the symptom development was caused by persistent "*Blood*" heat [4]. In TCM theory, the "*Lung*" governs "*Qi*" in the body, participating in the formation and movement of "*Qi*" originating from food nutrients and air breathes. On one hand, the "*Lung*" collects digested nutrients absorbed from the "*Spleen*" and "*Stomach*"; thereafter the "*Lung*" generates "*Blood*" through air exchange, as described in "*Lingshu Jing*" of "*Huangdi Neijing*" [4]. Under stress, "*Heat*" enters the "*Blood*" due to various factors, including the exogenous attack of pathogen and depressive emotion [4]. Thus, the etiology and pathogenesis of acne vulgaris can be explained by TCM theory, i.e. it is contributed by pathogenic and emotional factors. Another example is allergic urticaria appearing as pink or red itchy rashes on the skin. In "*Lingshu Jing*" of "*Huangdi Neijing*," abnormal seasonal weather had been proposed to weaken the human immune system, causing body shivering and hair erection under cold conditions, as well as perspiration from subcutaneous tissue. These responses are considered as a defense mechanism by the host in responding to external changes of environment, normally causing itchiness [4]. These historical records provide a foundation for formulation and development of cosmetics deriving from Chinese medicinal herbs.

2.3 THE HISTORICAL APPLICATION OF TCM IN COSMETOLOGY

In "*Zhongci Qijing*," of "*Classic of Mountains and Seas*" (400 BC), the herb *Ganoderma lucidum*, a reddish laccate species of *Ganoderma*, was first mentioned (as "*Yao Cao*"), possessing the function of promoting facial beauty [5]. In addition, the skincare application of herbal medicine can be chased back to the *Shang* dynasty (1600–1046 BC). The women of *Shang* applied the juice of *Carthamus tinctorius* (safflower) on their cheeks to make them look pink, which is the earliest blusher recorded in history. Despite the use of herbal medicine on skin, animal-derived product has been developed and applied for skin ameliorating functions. Porcine fat had been prepared in a paste and applied onto skin to facilitate wound healing, as recorded in "*Prescriptions for Fifty-Two Ailments*" (1065–771 BC) [6]. Aside from the medicinal form in paste for external application, other forms of skin cosmetics, e.g. by oral intake, had been developed and recorded in ancient literatures. For oral intake, TCM in the forms of decoction, tea, infusion, powder, or pill are tailored to enhance the pharmacological efficacy of active ingredients in serving as nutrients for skin. Herbal extracts could be in the form of cleanser, lotion, and paste for topical medication, steam bath, or hot compress therapies. Foot injuries caused by cold temperature could be cured by heat therapy. The injured foot was applied with ground onion, and thereafter the foot was warmed by a heated underground cavity, as described in "*Prescriptions for Fifty-Two Ailments*" [6]. Although the efficacy of Chinese herbs had not been scientifically indicated in most ancient literature, the principle of TCM has already been proposed and practiced in antiquity.

From 220 to 907 AD, the development of cosmetology in TCM grew rapidly. China had fallen into long term political instability, with continuous wars and frequent turnovers of regime. The formulation of TCM during this period was focused on the pharmacological efficacy and the cost of herbs. Also popular during this period was Taoism, in which alchemists had discovered the early techniques of herbal extraction and purification, as well as compound synthesis. The pursuit of an elixir by alchemists had helped the development of TCM formulation in treating disease, including skin problems.

In the Eastern Jin dynasty (226–420 AD), a well-known Chinese alchemist, Ge Hong had written a pocket size book, named "*Zhou Hou Bei Ji Fang.*" Over a hundred herbal formulas for skin application or treatment have been recorded in this book. The recorded herbal formulas included facial masks in promoting beauty, herbal sachets in eliminating body odor, and hair wax in polishing hair color. These historical records strengthen the knowledge of TCM in cosmetology. In the Tang dynasties (618–907 AD), great economic prosperity and deep cultural exchange among ethnic groups resulted from the establishment of international trading. Abundant TCM literatures emerged in this period, including the medicinal formulas from ethnic minorities. There are two important medicinal literatures from the Tang dynasty, written by a physician *Sun Simiao* (regarded as the king of medicine) and *Wang Dao*, "*Beiji Qianjin Yaofang*" and "*Waitai Miyao*," respectively: these two books documented numerous TCM formulas in improving and curing skin and/or hair diseases. The increasing usage of TCM for skin cosmetics reflected the popularity of personal makeup at that period.

The Song to Qing dynasty (960–1911 AD) marked the golden age of cosmetology in TCM application. TCM was officially valued by the local government, where an official pharmacy (the "*Taiping Benevolent Dispensary Bureau*") was established. The establishment of an official pharmacy had promoted the collection of ancient medicinal records and established the standardized production of herbal formulas. An important book in Chinese cosmetics, "*Tai Ping Sheng Hui Fang*," was written and published by the government bureau. Over a hundred herbal prescriptions were recorded in this book, and the popular prescription of "*Qi Bai Gao*" was first described. This prescription was recorded to be used commonly by concubines in the royal palace, with the objectives of removing freckles, soothing the skin, and preventing wrinkles through improving the "*Qi-Blood.*"

In the Jin and Yuan dynasties (1115–1355 AD), wars among various ethnic groups continued. Although this long period of war hindered the development of TCM in cosmetology, the appearance of four schools of thought in TCM provided academic arguments that revolutionized the theory and formulation of Chinese medicines. The four representative schools were: cold/cooling led by Liu Wansu, purgation led by Zhang Congzheng, spleen/stomach led by Li Dongyuen, and nourishing "Yin" led by Zhu Danxi. Taking skin allergy as an example, the cold/cooling school considered that skin itchiness and pain should be originated from "Heat" in "Zang-Fu," where slight "Heat" generated itchiness and subsequently severe "Heat" gave pain. According to the theory of Liu Wansu, the treatment principle of employing cold therapy should be recommended to relieve "Heat" or "Fire."

The purgation school of Zhang Congzheng believed that urticaria (hives) in babies originated from "Heat," accumulated before birth [7]. TCM practitioners inclined to the use of sweating, vomiting, and purgative therapies for treatment. The spleen/stomach school of Li Dongyuen proposed that terrestrial dampness attacked "Spleen" and "Stomach" causing skin diseases, and thus therapy to tonify "Qi" and "Blood" should be preferred [7]. The nourishing "Yin" school of Zhu Danxi interpreted that rashes were originated from "Heat" and phlegm, and should be remedied by eliminating "Lung" and "Fire" [8].

In the Ming to Qing dynasties (1368–1912 AD), the level of herbal formulas deriving from TCM reached a new height. In the early 15th century, the sea voyages of Zheng He visiting countries in the Western Pacific and Indian oceans brought foreign cosmetic herbs into China, e.g. Boswellia carterii (frankincense or olibanum-tree), Benzoinum styracis (Sumatra benzoin tree), and Liquidambar orientalis (Oriental sweet gum). During the Ming dynasty, two important medicinal literatures were published by Zhu Su and Li Shizhen ("Pu Ji Fang" and "Compendium of Materia Medica," respectively). In these two books over a thousand cosmetics formulas had been record, many of them tailored for facial beauty. After the opium wars (1839–1860 AD), Western medicines emerged into China with the establishment of medical schools by missionaries and doctors. These new interactions had facilitated the combination of Chinese and Western medicines in cosmetology, which subsequently led to the booming of modern TCM cosmetics.

2.4 THE COSMETIC FUNCTION OF TCM

Skin pigmentation is mainly caused by UV exposure, in which melanin synthesis happens as a protective mechanism against UV damage. Melanin synthesis in dermal melanocytes is the major cause of skin pigmentation.

During this process the central enzyme, tyrosinase, triggers the oxidation of L-tyrosine to dopaquinone. This leads to the synthesis of two major types of melanin: eumelanin and pheomelanin, causing skin darkening [9]. Skin lightening agents have been developed to address the concerns of consumers to improve their complexion. Especially in Asia, women tend to have a negative perception towards dark skin, and pale skin is considering beautiful. From the perspective of TCM, there have been a great number of herbs or extracts demonstrating a positive effect in promoting skin fairness. For examples, pearl powder, from natural pearls, is beneficial to promoting skin glossiness, according to ancient Chinese literatures. The earliest record about pearl powder prescribed in skin whitening treatment can be traced back to the Ming Dynasty (1578 AD), by Li Shizhen in "*Compendium of Materia Medica*", stating that "applying the pearl to the face can make the skin moisturized and glossy." Pearl powder is rich in nutrients and contains calcium carbonates, proteins, and short peptides [10]. In enzymatic assay, pearl extract inhibited the activity of tyrosinase in converting L-tyrosine to dopaquinone [11], supporting the description in TCM literatures.

Many herbs have been identified as potential whitening agents, as they are able to inhibit the activity of tyrosinase and the subsequent melanin synthesis. *Gentiana veitchiorum* (Chinese gentian) is a common TCM herb with anti-microbial, anti-inflammatory, hepatoprotective, and anti-oxidative functions [12–14]. The extract of *G. veitchiorum* flowers was able to downregulate melanin synthesis in cultured melanocytes by suppressing the transcription of melanogenic enzymes, i.e. tyrosinase, tyrosinase-related protein 1 and tyrosinase-related protein 2, as well as suppressing the master transcription factor (i.e. MITF) of these enzymes [15] (Figure 2.1). In addition, other TCM herbs

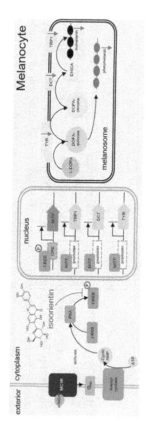

FIGURE 2.1 The proposed action of *Gentiana veitchiorum* in anti-melanin production. The flower of *G. veitchiorum* contains isoorientin that suppresses melanin production through downregulation of tyrosinase, tyrosinase-related proteins, microphthalmia-associated transcription factor (MITF), and inhibition of cAMP response element-binding protein (CREB) phosphorylation. This implies that the flower of *G. veitchiorum* may be a naturally occurring skin de-pigmenting agent.

or formulae have been identified to have tyrosinase-inhibiting effects, including the herbs of *Polygonum cuspidatum* (Japanese knotweed) and *Ampelopsis japonica* (Japanese pepper vine), and the herbal formulae of *Qian-wang-hong-bai-san* and *Qiong-yu-gao* [16]. The findings illustrate that many potential whitening agents can be developed from TCM herbs.

Oxidative stress is attributing to skin aging, manifested by altered skin contour, wrinkling, pigmented spots and facial sagging [17]. The source of oxidative stress could be intrinsic or extrinsic; the former is genetically determined, while the latter one is mainly UV- and toxic exposure-mediated, e.g. by sunlight, smoking, and alcohol consumption [18]. A natural anti-aging agent would work by inhibiting or down-regulating oxidative stress, i.e. reducing reactive oxygen species (ROS). There are a few TCM herbs that have strong anti-oxidative functions, such as *Panax ginseng* (Chinese/Korean ginseng), *Astragalus membranaceus* var. *mongholicus* or *A. membranaceus* (milkvetch plant), and *Coix lacryma-joni* L. var. *mayuen* (Coix seed) [19]. As a support for TCM for skin anti-aging, different doses of water extracts deriving from *Codonopsis pilosula* var. *modesta* (Codonopsis) have been prescribed to D-galactose-induced aging mice [20]. The intake of herbal extract in aging mice was able to suppress lipid peroxidation, i.e. malondialdehyde and lipofuscin, which up-regulated the activity of anti-oxidative enzymes [21]. Again, Codonopsis is a well-known antioxidant in TCM.

An accumulation of collagen breakdown is also regarded as one important factor in aging skin, leading to weakened mechanical tension and subsequently wrinkles. There are two types of collagen in human skin – type I and III collagen; the former is found predominantly in adult human skin, and type III collagen predominates in fetal tissue [22]. In aged women, a decrease in these two types of collagen in dermis has been demonstrated [22]. Thus, TCM herbs or compounds, in boosting the production of collagen or slowing down the breakdown of collagen, should help in the search of anti-aging agents. In this scenario, phytoestrogens derived from TCM herbs or from vegetables have been found to have functions in anti-aging, especially in up-regulating collagen contents. The functions of these phytoestrogens are mediated by estrogenic signaling [4]. This anti-aging phytochemical can be exemplified by resveratrol, a common flavonoid derived from Chinese herbs, e.g. *P. cuspidatum* (Japanese knotweed) or from grapes [23]. In animal studies, the intake of resveratrol could increase collagen synthesis and inhibit collagen degradation, triggered by matrix metalloproteinases (MMPs) by stimulating tissue inhibitor of metalloproteinases (TIMPl); the eventual outcome was to promote the production of skin collagen [24, 25]. In addition, an anti-aging effect has been identified from the essential oil of *Angelicae sinensis* (known as female ginseng) in the human dermal fibroblast cell model, which could increase the secretion of type I collagen.

2.5 THE ACTIVE INGREDIENTS OF TCM IN COSMETOLOGY

Phytochemicals from TCM herbs suggested as responsible for activity in skin cosmetics can be mainly categorized into polyphenol, saponin, and alkaloid [26]. Each kind of phytochemicals has been identified as having different functions in improving skin condition and thus having potential to be applied in a cosmetic product. Polyphenols are naturally synthesized in the secondary metabolism of plants, including flavonoids and non-flavonoids, i.e. phenolic acids, lignans, and stilbenes [27]. The known health benefits of polyphenols as nutraceuticals include anti-oxidation, anti-inflammation, and immunomodulation [28]. Several lines of evidence have suggested their functions in modulating skin cells. Resveratrol has a broad spectrum of properties, e.g. anti-aging, skin whitening, and anti-acne [25]. It protects skin against UVA radiation in keratinocytes, which counters photoaging by decreasing free radicals, as well as preventing lipid oxidation. In addition, resveratrol modulates tyrosinase activity by inhibiting the expression of melanogenesis-related enzymes and the master transcription factor MITF in human melanocytes [25, 29]. Isoorientin, a flavonoid from *G. veitchiorum* has shown inhibitory effect on melanin production through suppressing the cyclic adenosine monophosphate (cAMP) signaling pathway (Figure 2.1), which subsequently could down-regulate the expression of melanogenic enzymes, resulted in a decrease of melanin synthesis in skin [30].

Ginsenoside, a well-known TCM saponin from ginseng [31], has been shown to act as a therapeutic option for skin photoaging and injury [32]. The mechanistic studies of ginsenosides showed the regulation of p38 mitogen-activated protein kinases (MAPK)/MSK2/nuclear factor kappa-light-chain-enhancer of activated B cells (NF-κB) signaling in skin dermal fibroblast during wound healing [33]. Moreover, the effect of ginsenoside in preventing hair loss has been well recognized, and indeed which has been widely applied in several hair or scalp treatment products commercially.

TCM alkaloids have been shown to be skin regulators; caffeine is the best-known example. By activating autophagy, caffeine could ameliorate the oxidative stress-induced senescence and abnormal aging [34]. In addition, caffeine has been characterized as a photo-protectant against the impact of UV radiation to hair and scalp health [15]. Sinomenine, an alkaloid derived from *Sinomenium acutum* (Tsuzurafuji) could suppress the lipopolysaccharides (LPS)-induced inflammation by reducing CCAT1 expression in skin keratinocytes [34]. Capsaicin, the major ingredient in chili pepper, inhibited the melanin content in melanocytes and skin. Capsaicin activates the transient receptor potential cation channel subfamily V member 1 (TRPV1) and the Ca^{2+} mobilization, leading to a down-regulation of the melanogenic enzymes [35].

2.6 THE PERSPECTIVE OF TCM IN DEVELOPING COSMETIC PRODUCTS

Today, the consumers of cosmetic products pay more attention to the processing methods and ingredients being used in the products. This phenomenon is known as "green beauty," in which the consumers tend to purchase cosmetic goods that are natural or organic. Due to this trend, global skincare brands launch cosmetic products that are claimed to be chemical-free and natural. From the market research conducted by Premium Beauty Media and Future Market Insights (FMI), the global market value for natural cosmetics and personal care from 2018 to 2027 is expected to be about US$20 billion in 10 years' time.

Cosmetic products deriving from Chinese herbs have been launched, e.g. *Angelica dahurica* (Dahurian angelica), *Typhonium giganteum* (Chinese aroid), and *Poria cocos* (Poria mushroom) [19] (Table 2.1). To meet market need, the TCM-deriving skincare products have attracted lots of attention recently, not just in Asian societies but also in Western countries. In the application of TCM in cosmetics, the product is based on either TCM theories or TCM active ingredients, to achieve different skincare functions. In view of the increasing demand for natural cosmetics, the future of TCM in cosmetic products should be positive. However, the action mechanism and active ingredient within a TCM herb are often not fully resolved, which hinders future development. This obstacle of providing scientific evidence to support the cosmetic functions of TCM therefore has to be resolved.

As the supply of TCM in cosmetic products exceeds demand, measures must be taken to improve the source of TCM materials. There are two critical problems in TCM herbs: quality control and contamination of toxic substance. According to the World Health Organization, the adulteration of herbal products is a common problem that threatens the safety of consumers. The expensive herb, or a better grading herb, is frequently mixed with cheaper herbs, or even different species of herb, as the final products, which eventually reduces the efficacy, and in many cases causes safety concerns. Another common problem in supplying TCM materials is the contamination with heavy metal, e.g. chromium, copper, zinc, lead, mercury, as well as insecticide. These problems are now being resolved by practicing good agriculture and collection

TABLE 2.1   TCM in cosmetic application

TCM	FUNCTION	SOURCE
Ganoderma lucidum	Adjusting skin color	Classic of Mountains and Seas[a]
Carthamus tinctorius	Adjusting skin color	Prescriptions for Fifty-Two Ailments[b]
Porcine fat	Wound healing	[2]
Heat therapy	Cold injury	Prescriptions for Fifty-Two Ailments
Qi Bai Gao[c]	Remove freckles, soothe skin and prevent wrinkles	Tai Ping Sheng Hui Fang[d]
Pearl powder	Skin lightening	Compendium of Materia Medica[e]
Edible bird nest	Skin lightening	[10]
Gentiana veitchiorum	Skin lightening	[30]
Polygonum cuspidatum	Skin lightening	[16]
Ampelopsis japonica	Skin lightening	[27]
Capsicum chinense	Skin lightening	[35]
Panax ginseng	Anti-skin aging	
Astragalus membranaceus	Anti-skin aging	[22]
Coix lacryma-joni	Anti-skin aging	[22]
Angelica dahurica	Skin lightening and anti-acne	[22]
Rhizoma typhonii	Skin lightening and anti-acne	[22]
Poria cocos	Anti-skin aging	[22]
Polygonum cuspidatum	Skin lightening	[22]
Ampelopsis japonica	Skin lightening	[16]
Qian Wang Hong Bai San[f]	Skin lightening	[16]
Qiong Yu Gao[g]	Skin lightening	[16]
Codonopsis pilosula	Suppress lipid peroxidation	[21]

[a] Record in Zhongci Qijing, 400 BC.
[b] Written 1065–771 BC.
[c] A prescription to remove freckles, soothe skin and prevent wrinkles.
[d] A cosmetic book written by "Taiping Benevolent Dispensary Bureau."
[e] Written by Li Shizhen in the Ming Dynasty, 1578 AD.
[f] An ancient Chinese herbal formula, used as a skin whitening agent.
[g] A popular Chinese herbal formula, described 840 years ago.

practice (GACP) farming in China. However, problems still frequently occur. The farming and preparation of TCM should follow the specific requirements of pharmacopoeia, including Chinese and/or European pharmacopoeia.

TCM in cosmetics products are not only in China only but show potential to enter the global market. Industries seek an opportunity to promote their brands and products to the huge Chinese market, which can generate billions of dollars in revenue. The increasing attention and popularity of TCM cosmetics, as well as the China cosmetic market, are attracting overseas industries to take this opportunity.

REFERENCES

1. Yu CC, Liang JZ (2016). The functions of componential analysis to the translation of cultural animal images in the Classic of Mountains and Seas. Sino-US English Teaching, 13, 724–735.
2. Hou J, Kim S (2018). Possible role of ginsenoside Rb1 in skin wound healing via regulating senescent skin dermal fibroblast. Biochemical and Biophysical Research Communications, 499, 381–388.
3. Chaudhri SK, Jain NK (2009). History of cosmetics. Asian Journal of Pharmaceutics, 3, 164–167.
4. Zhang ZF, Yuan LIU, Lu-Yang LU, et al. (2014). Hepatoprotective activity of Gentiana veitchiorum Hemsl. against carbon tetrachloride-induced hepatotoxicity in mice. Chinese Journal of Natural Medicines, 12, 488–494.
5. Wu QY, Wong ZCF, Wang C, et al. (2019). Isoorientin derived from Gentiana veitchiorum Hemsl. flowers inhibits melanogenesis by down-regulating MITF-induced tyrosinase expression. Phytomedicine, 57, 129–136.
6. Lephart ED (2017). Resveratrol, 4′ acetoxy resveratrol, R-equol, racemic equol or S-equol as cosmeceuticals to improve dermal health. International Journal of Molecular Sciences, 18, 1193.
7. Wu QY, Bai PZ, Xia YT, et al. (2020). Capsaicin inhibits the expression of melanogenic proteins in melanocyte via activation of TRPV1 channel: identifying an inhibitor of skin melanogenesis. Journal of Agricultural and Food Chemistry, 68, 14863–14873.
8. Zhang CZ (1999). Ru Men Shi Qin (1st ed., Chinese Materia Medica; Vol. 238). Beijing: Huaxia Publishing House.
9. Liu Y, Zhao C, Ma Q, et al. (2019). Sinomenine retards LPS-elicited inflammation via down-regulating CCAT1 in HaCaT cells. Life Sciences, 233, 116703.
10. Chan GKL, Wong, ZCF, Lam KYC, Cheng LKW, Zhang LM, Lin H, Dong TT, Tsim KWK (2015). Edible bird's nest, an Asian health food supplement, possesses skin lightening activities: identification of N-acetylneuraminic acid as active ingredient. Journal of Cosmetics, Dermatological Sciences and Applications, 5, 262.
11. Huang F, Parker R, Cui H (2011). Cosmetology in Chinese Medicine. PMPH: USA.

12. Herrmann F, Wink M (2011). Synergistic interactions of saponins and monoterpenes in HeLa cells, Cos7 cells and in erythrocytes. Phytomedicine, 18, 1191–1196.

13. Liu C (2016). Review on the studies of unearthed Mawangdui medical books. Chinese Studies, 5, 6–14.

14. Ye Y, Chou GX, Mu DD, et al. (2010). Screening of Chinese herbal medicines for anti-tyrosinase activity in a cell free system and B16 cells. Journal of Ethnopharmacology, 129, 387–390.

15. Chen X, Peng LH, Chee SS, et al. (2019). Nano-scaled pearl powder accelerates wound repair and regeneration *in vitro* and *in vivo*. Drug Development and Industrial Pharmacy, 45, 1009–1016.

16. Wu C, Hou Q, Hu F, et al. (2014). Effect of Suhua Codonopsis on antioxidant capacity of D-galactose-induced aging mice. Pharmacology and Clinics of Chinese Medicine, 30, 92–96.

17. Pillaiyar T, Manickam M, Jung SH (2017). Downregulation of melanogenesis: drug discovery and therapeutic options. Drug Discovery Today, 22, 282–298.

18. Newton RA, Cook AL, Roberts DW, et al. (2007). Post-transcriptional regulation of melanin biosynthetic enzymes by cAMP and resveratrol in human melanocytes. The Journal of Investigative Dermatology, 127, 2216–2227.

19. Sabouri-Rad S, Sabouri-Rad S, Sahebkar A, et al. (2017). Ginseng in dermatology: a review. Current Pharmaceutical Design, 23, 1649–1666.

20. Rinnerthaler M, Bischof J, Streubel MK, et al. (2015). Oxidative stress in aging human skin. Biomolecules, 5, 545–589.

21. Umbayev B, Askarova, S, Almabayeva A, et al. (2020). Galactose-induced skin aging: the role of oxidative stress. Oxidative Medicine and Cellular Longevity, 2020, 1–15.

22. Liu, P., Zhao, H. Luo, Y (2017) Anti-aging implications of *Astragalus membranaceus* (Huangqi): a well-known Chinese tonic. Aging and Disease, 8, 868.

23. Hwang HJ, Hung CH (2010). Comparison of hydration, tyrosinase resistance, and antioxidant activation in three kinds of pearl powders. Journal of Cosmetic Science, 61, 133–145.

24. Gherardini J, Wegner J, Chéret J, et al. (2019). Trans-epidermal UV radiation of scalp skin *ex vivo* induces hair follicle damage that is alleviated by the topical treatment with caffeine. International Journal of Cosmetic Science, 41, 164–182.

25. Mrduljaš N, Krešić G, Bilušić T (2017). Polyphenols: food sources and health benefits. In Functional Food-Improve Health through Adequate Food. In Tech Open.

26. Ratz-Łyko A, Arct J (2019). Resveratrol as an active ingredient for cosmetic and dermatological applications: a review. Journal of Cosmetic and Laser Therapy, 21, 84–90.

27. Leu, YL, Hwang, TL, Hu, JW, Fang, JY (2008) Anthraquinones from *Polygonum cuspidatum* as tyrosinase inhibitors for dermal use. Phytotherapy Research, 22, 552–556.

28. Liu C, Yang S, Wang K, et al. (2019). Alkaloids from traditional Chinese medicine against hepatocellular carcinoma. Biomedicine & Pharmacotherapy, 120, 109543.

29. Liu WS (1967). Huangdi Su Wen Xuanming Lun Fang. Taibei: Yi Wen.

30. Wang KH, Lin RD, Hsu FL, et al. (2006). Cosmetic applications of selected traditional Chinese herbal medicines. Journal of Ethnopharmacology, 106(3), 353–359.

31. Giardina S, Michelotti A, Zavattini G, et al. (2010). Efficacy study *in vitro*: assessment of the properties of resveratrol and resveratrol+ *N*-acetylcysteine on proliferation and inhibition of collagen activity. Minerva Ginecologica, 62, 195–201.

32. Poljšak B, Dahmane RG, Godić A (2012). Intrinsic skin aging: the role of oxidative stress. Acta Dermatovenerol Alp Pannonica Adriats, 21, 33–36.

33. Hou Y, Cao W, Li T, et al. (2011). *Gentiana veitchiorum* particles inhibited LPS induced pulmonary alveolar macrophages (AM) TNF-α production and the underlying mechanism. Chinese Journal of Cellular and Molecular Immunology, 27, 364–366.

34. Li YF, Ouyang SH, Tu LF, et al. (2018). Caffeine protects skin from oxidative stress-induced senescence through the activation of autophagy. Theranostics, 8, 5713–5730.

35. Williams HC, Dellavalle RP, Garner S (2012). Acne vulgaris. The Lancet, 379, 361–372.

3

In vitro and *in vivo* Assessments of Phytocosmetics in Skin Care

Yushi Katsuyama and Hitoshi Masaki

Contents

3.1 INTRODUCTION

The skin is an important organ giving an initial perspective and impression regarding our health and age. Thus, keeping the skin healthy and beautiful by skin care is often considered an important component to a fulfilling life.

Human beings carry out skin care to achieve the following purposes: moisturizing to keep the skin healthy and reducing pigmented spots and wrinkles to make the skin look young and beautiful. Phenomena such as pigmented spots and wrinkles regarding skin aging are initiated and accelerated by excessive reactive oxygen species (ROS). In fact, many reports have shown that antioxidants have beneficial effects to prevent and/or improve skin aging.

Here we introduce the mechanisms involved in the intracellular and extracellular production of ROS, and the relationships with skin dryness and the appearance of pigmented spots and wrinkles. We then introduce methods used to assess phytochemicals and products formulated to treat those phenomena, according to the mechanisms involved.

3.2 ANTI-OXIDATION

3.2.1 Concept of Anti-Oxidation

Our skin is exposed daily to sunlight, which contains ultraviolet (UV) radiation. Thus, it is hard to discuss maintaining or improving skin conditions while ignoring the influence of sunlight. Among the various wavelengths in sunlight, UV is a strong generator of ROS and reactive nitrogen species (RNS) in the epidermis and dermis [1]. For instance, superoxide anion radicals ($\cdot O_2^-$) and nitric oxide radicals ($NO\cdot$) are generated in skin resident cells, keratinocytes and fibroblasts irradiated with UV through enzymatic reactions such as NADPH oxidase and nitric oxide synthase (NOS), respectively [2, 3]. Those radicals dysregulate skin functions related to skin beauty due to the accumulation of carbonylated proteins (CPs) [4] and the nitration of tyrosine residues in proteins [5]. On the other hand, cells in our skin synthesize anti-oxidative enzymes and substances, such as catalase and glutathione (GSH), through the NF-E2-related factor 2 (Nrf2)-anti-oxidant response element (ARE) pathway to protect against intracellular ROS and RNS [6]. However, levels of those substances are decreased following single or chronic UV exposures and with age, resulting in increased intracellular oxidation conditions.

To maintain or improve skin conditions for health and beauty, the first step is to minimize the skin's exposure to oxidation conditions and the approach is to directly scavenge ROS and/or enhance the intracellular anti-oxidant system.

3.2.2 The Anti-Oxidation Effects of Phytochemicals

Jixueteng, the dried stem of *Spatholobus suberectus* Dunn (Leguminosae), is a traditional Chinese herbal medicine. *Jixueteng* water extracts show scavenging activity against ·OH and ·O_2^-, and those effects were stronger than co-enzyme Q10, a well-known antioxidant assessed by electron spin resonance (ESR) [7]. *Jixueteng* contains various components, predominantly polyphenols including flavonoids that are responsible for their effects of ROS scavenging. The green leaves of *Camellia japonica* (CJGL) show a scavenging activity against -OH and H_2O_2 in chemical studies. Also, in biological studies, CJGL suppressed intracellular ROS levels in keratinocytes [8]. Furthermore, CJGL reduced CP levels in tape-stripped stratum corneum (SC) after UVB irradiation. These results suggested that natural extracts with the ability to scavenge ROS directly have the potential to suppress intracellular oxidative levels and protect from the accumulation of CPs in the SC.

Agastache rugosa Kuntze, used as a traditional herbal medicine against photoaging, attenuated ROS generation induced by UVB through the enhancement of GSH synthesis and superoxide dismutase (SOD) activity in keratinocytes [9]. Ginger phenylpropanoids and quercetin increased glutathione-S-transferase through the activation of Nrf2 signaling in keratinocytes and fibroblasts [10]. Thus, some traditional plant extracts exert anti-oxidation effects through the activation of the intracellular anti-oxidation system.

3.2.3 Assays for Anti-Oxidant Potential

3.2.3.1 ROS scavenging assay by electron spin resonance (ESR)

The scavenging of ROS can be directly measured using the ESR spin-trapping method. That technique can detect each type of radical as follows:

- ·O_2^- detection: [11] ·O_2^-, generated by the enzymatic reaction of xanthine oxidase and hypoxanthine, is spin-trapped with 5,5-dimethyl-1-pyrroline 1-oxide.
- NO-detection: [12] NO, generated with 1-hydroxy-2-oxo-3-(*N*-methyl-3-aminopropyl)-3-methyl-1-triazene (NOC-7), is spin-trapped with 2-(4-carboxyphenyl)-4,4,5,5-tetramethylimidazoline-1-oxyl-3-oxide, sodium salt (cPTIO).

3.2.3.2 Determination of intracellular ROS levels [13]

Intracellular ROS levels are determined using 2′,7′-dichlorodihydrofluorescein diacetate.

3.2.3.3 Determination of intracellular CP levels in monolayer cells and in corneocytes [8, 14, 15]

CPs in cells and corneocytes are fluorescence-labeled with 20 µM fluorescein-5-thiosemicarbazine. Fluorescence images are captured using a fluorescence microscope. CP levels in corneocytes are quantified in each fluorescence image using corneocytometry software (CIEL, Tokyo, Japan).

3.2.3.4 Evaluation of Nrf2-ARE signaling

Immunostaining analysis of the translocation of Nrf2 [13,16]: After fixing cells with 4% formaldehyde, nonspecific binding is blocked by treatment with 1% IgG-free bovine serum albumin (BSA). An anti-Nrf2 antibody is used for immunofluorescent staining, and a secondary antibody is used to label antibodies that have bound to Nrf2. Nuclei of cells are stained with 2 µM Hoechst 33342.

3.3 SKIN MOISTURIZING

3.3.1 Concept of Skin Moisturizing

Water in the SC is maintained by the integration of two functions, the water holding function and the barrier function. The water holding function of the SC is exhibited by natural moisturizing factor (NMF), composed of free amino acids, pyrrolidonecarboxylic acid (PCA), lactic acid, urea and metals. On the other hand, the barrier function of the SC is exhibited by several substances and mechanisms such as sebum, corneocytes, the intercellular lamellar structure of lipids containing ceramide and tight junctions.

Regarding the relationship between ROS and moisturizing, extracellular H_2O_2 down-regulates the messenger RNA (mRNA) expression of serine palmitoyl transferase (SPT), the rate-limiting enzyme of ceramide synthesis [17]. GSH depletion of reconstructed human epidermal equivalents (RHEEs) by treatment with buthionine sulfoximine, leading to higher intracellular ROS levels, produces immature corneocytes through the reduced protein expression level of transglutaminase-1 (TGM-1) [18].

In conclusion, ROS produces an immature SC, which has a lower barrier function through the adverse modulation of the terminal differentiation of keratinocytes.

3.3.2 Characteristics of Dry Skin which is Less Moisturizing

Dry skin is characterized as skin that has lower water content at the surface and a higher rate of water evaporation from the surface (TEWL; trans-epidermal water loss) due to dysfunction of the water holding and barrier functions. The SC of dry skin shows a higher ratio of interleukin (IL)-1α receptor antagonist (RA) and IL-1α (IL-1αRA/IL-1α) [19] and contains CPs at a higher frequency [20]. In an *in vitro* study reproducing dry skin, it has been demonstrated that exposure of RHEEs to low humidity at the SC causes the excess generation of ROS and the secretion of IL-1α [21].

In conclusion, it is considered that dry skin is in a higher oxidation condition according to inflammation.

3.3.3 The Effects of Phytochemicals on Skin Moisturizing and the Skin Barrier

Treatment with a Eucalyptus extract increased the levels of ceramide in keratinocytes and in RHEEs, which resulted from the activated synthesis of ceramide, glucosylceramide and sphingomyelin through the up-regulation of the mRNA expression levels of the enzymes involved [22]. Interestingly, application of the Eucalyptus extract on dry skin for 28 days recovered the water holding and barrier functions of the SC due to the improved ceramide profile of the SC [23]. Niacinamide, also known as vitamin B₃, not only suppressed the oxidative stress induced by UV irradiation and external stimuli, but also increased ceramide contents due to the normalization of skin turnover [24]. In a UV challenge clinical trial, pretreatment with 5% niacinamide reduced erythema and the IL-1 increased ceramide contents [25].

3.3.4 Mechanisms Regarding Skin Moisture

3.3.4.1 Water holding function

Free amino acids: Filaggrin, a precursor protein of the free amino acids in NMF, is biosynthesized as profilaggrin in differentiated keratinocytes at the upper spinous cell layer. Profilaggrin is stored in keratohyalin granules in granular cells. Filaggrin is generated from profilaggrin by cleavage with proteases such as calpain, furin, etc [26]. The important role of filaggrin is to assemble keratin filaments into bundles in corneocytes. Once filaggrin has completed that role, it is further degraded to amino acids by calpain, caspase 14 and bleomycin hydrolase [26].

3.3.4.2 Barrier function

Corneocytes: Corneocytes are terminally differentiated keratinocytes critical to the barrier function of the SC since they physically cover the surface of the human body. Corneocytes have a cornified cell envelope (CE), composed of involucrin, loricrin, filaggrin and small proline rich protein [27], and a cornified lipid envelope (CLE), formed by covalent bonding with ceramides, at the outside of the CE [28]. The CE provides strong resistance against chemicals, and the CLE provides hydrophobicity and serves as a scaffold for spreading lipid lamellar sheets at interstices between corneocytes. The CE and CLE are formed by transglutaminases through cross-links between glutamines and lysines in component proteins [29] and esterifications between terminal carboxylic acids in involucrin and hydroxyl groups at the ω-position of ceramides [30].

Lamellar structure of intercellular lipids: Lipid lamellar sheets, assembled by ceramides, cholesterol and free fatty acids are located stacked at the interstices of corneocytes [31]. Ceramides are synthesized by serine palmitoyl transferase and ceramide synthases [32].

Tight junctions: Tight junctions are composed of occludin-1, claudin-1 and zona occludens protein-1, and act as a reversible gate for metal ions and water at the second layer of the granular cell layer [33].

3.3.5 Assays for Skin Moisturizing Functions

3.3.5.1 Evaluation of skin barrier function using RHEES [17]

RHEEs (LabCyte EPI-MODEL 6D, Japan Tissue Engineering, Aichi, Japan) are topically treated with samples on their SC and are then cultivated for a suitable number of days. The skin barrier function is evaluated by measuring TEWL with a handy TEWL measuring instrument (VAPO SCAN AS-VT100RS, Asahi Techno Lab, Yokohama, Japan). Ceramides in RHEEs are determined using high-performance thin-layer chromatography (HPTLC, Merck, Darmstadt, Germany) with chloroform: methanol: acetic acid = 190: 9: 1 (v/v) as a development solvent.

3.3.5.2 In vivo assay using tape-stripped corneocytes [15, 19, 34]

Skin conditions are estimated by measuring various parameters originating from corneocytes. The size of corneocytes reflects the turnover rate of the SC. If the size of corneocytes becomes smaller, it indicates that the turnover rate of the SC has become faster. The degree of thick abrasion shows the degree of skin dryness. The maturity of corneocytes is determined according to the ratio of the status of the CE and CLE. The CE status is measured by the loss of immunoreactivity with involucrin obtained by immunostaining with the corresponding antibody, and the CLE status is estimated by the fluorescence intensity of corneocytes treated with Nile red. As a biological parameter of inflammation in the epidermis, the ratio of IL-1 RA and IL-1α is measured using an enzyme-linked immunosorbent assay (ELISA).

3.4 PIGMENTATION

3.4.1 Concept of Pigmentation

Pigmented spots that appear at restricted areas on the skin surface are classified as freckles, solar lentigos (SLs) and melasma. SLs are the most common type of pigmented spots appearing on the skin depending on its history of sun exposure and its phototype [35] and are important targets for cosmetics. The characteristic feature of the epidermis at regions of SLs is thickening, the development of rete ridges [35, 36] and alterations of the dermal-epidermal junction such as the loss of heparan sulfate [37]. Furthermore, fibroblasts with a senescent phenotype are present in the dermis under SLs [38].

In general, pigmented spots on the surface of the skin result from the following processes; first, the excess synthesis of melanin in melanosomes (MSs) in melanocytes, and second, the diffusion of MSs filled with melanin through their transfer from melanocytes to keratinocytes. In fact, it has been recently demonstrated that the appearance of pigmented spots progresses due to undesirable communications between keratinocytes, fibroblasts and melanocytes triggered by UV irradiation and excessive levels of ROS [39–41]. "Substances involved in communication from keratinocytes to melanocytes include α-melanocyte stimulating hormone (α-MSH), stem cell factor (SCF), endothelin-1 and prostaglandin E_2 (PGE_2) [42–45]. Meanwhile, fibroblasts activate melanocytes through their secretion of various factors, including hepatocyte growth factor (HGF), keratinocyte growth factor (KGF)/fibroblast growth factor-7 (FGF-7) and SCF. Fibroblasts also supply messages that can inactivate melanocytes such as dickkopf-related protein 1 (DKK-1) and stromal cell-derived factor 1 (SDF-1) [38].

In conclusion, although it is currently known that the activity of melanocytes is modulated by substances secreted from keratinocytes and fibroblasts, other important contributors may be identified by future studies.

3.4.2 The Anti-Pigmentation Effects of Phytochemicals

Madecassoside (MA) isolated from *Centella asiatica* (L.) inhibits UVR-induced melanin synthesis in a keratinocyte–melanocyte co-culture system and in in vivo assays [46]. Since MA suppresses the production of PGE_2 and PAR-2 in keratinocytes, it inhibits the elongation of dendrites in melanocytes and the incorporation of MSs into keratinocytes. Also, MA significantly decreases melanin content in RHEEs exposed to UVB or treated with SLIGRL, an agonist of PAR-2. In an in vivo study, topical application of 0.05% MA on the skin significantly reduced the UV-induced melanin index. An extract of red pumpkin seed (RPS; *Cucurbita maxima*), a special crop in Kanayama-machi in Japan, suppressed the incorporation of fluorescent beads (used as pseudo-MSs) into keratinocytes due to the activation of Nrf2 signaling [16].

Thus, the suppression of oxidative stress in keratinocytes can be considered an effective approach to improve pigmentation without the risk of hypopigmented skin such as vitiligo.

3.4.3 Assays for UVB-Induced Pigmentation

3.4.3.1 Melanocyte proliferation in conditioned medium prepared from UVB-irradiated keratinocytes [47]

After UVB irradiation, keratinocytes are cultured in fresh medium for 24 h and the medium is used as UVB-irradiated keratinocyte-conditioned medium (NHEK CM). Normal human epidermal melanocytes (NHEMs) are cultured with the UVB-irradiated NHEK CM for 24 h and their proliferation is quantified using the MTT assay.

3.4.3.2 Incorporation of MSs into keratinocytes cultured with NHEK CM [16]

NHEKs are cultured with a cocktail of NHEK CM and fluorescent beads (FluoSpheres® carboxylate-modified 0.2 µm, blue, Invitrogen) used as pseudo-MSs. The incorporation of fluorescent beads is quantified by measuring the fluorescence of the cell lysates.

3.4.3.3 Melanogenesis in RHEEs

The effects of phytochemicals on melanin production are examined using RHEEs containing melanocytes, commercially available from MatTek life science (Ashland, MA, USA). Phytochemicals are applied to RHEEs from the upper side, which are then cultured in the specified medium for a suitable number of days. Melanogenesis in RHEEs is estimated by measuring the L* value or by colorimetric quantification of melanin after solubilization by boiling in NaOH.

3.4.3.4 In vivo assay of anti-UV-induced pigmentation

The *in vivo* anti-pigmentation effects are evaluated by the suppression or lightening of UV-induced skin pigmentation. The pigmentation is stimulated by a single (1.8 MED to 2.0 MED) or multiple (0.8 MED to 1 MED) irradiations with solar simulated-UV light. The degree of pigmentation is evaluated by differences of L* value measured with a spectrometer between pre-irradiation and post-irradiation, or between non-irradiated sites and irradiated sites.

3.5 ANTI-WRINKLE EFFECTS ON PHOTOAGED SKIN

3.5.1 Concept of Photoaging

Since wrinkles are typical characteristics of skin aging that are accelerated by chronic sun exposure; that type of skin aging is termed photoaging in contrast to chronological aging. In general, it is recognized that wrinkles are caused by structural alterations of the dermal matrix, especially in the papillary dermis. The characteristic feature of the papillary dermal structure in sun-exposed elderly skin include a disrupted basement membrane [48], reduced numbers of collagen fibers [49] and the loss of fine elastic fibers, oxytalan fibers [50].

On the other hand, in the reticular dermis, the number of elastin fibers parallel in the skin or are non-oriented is increased [50], a symptom termed solar elastosis.

3.5.1.1 Depletion of collagen fibers

Type I collagen is the dominant structural component in the dermis and plays a critical role in maintaining the mechanical strength of the skin [51]. It is recognized that collagen synthesis is regulated by TGF-β-Smad signaling [52] and is suppressed by CCN-1/Cyr61, and that the degradation of collagen fibers is initiated by matrix metalloproteinase-1 (MMP-1) [53]. ROS is a critical trigger in collagen depletion due to its reduction of collagen synthesis and its acceleration of collagen degradation. ROS leads to the synthesis of AP-1 (activator protein 1), a heterodimer of c-Jun and c-Fos, through the activation of EGF-JNK signaling and NF-κB-ERK1/2 signaling, respectively [54, 55]. AP-1 enhances the biosynthesis of CCN-1/Cyr61 and MMP-1 through the upregulation of their mRNA expression levels.

3.5.1.2 Disappearance of oxytalan fibers

Elastic fibers are complicated structures due to their assembly with the assistance of several proteins [56]. The basic structure of elastic fibers is that tropoelastin adheres to microfibrils which are assembled from fibrillin-1and fibrillin-2. Tropoelastin adheres to the elastin microfibril interface located protein 1 of microfibrils with the assistance of fibulin-4 and fibulin-5, and finally is fixed on microfibrils due to cross-linking by lysyl oxidase. However, the assembly process and the assistance of member proteins of elastic fibers have not been fully elucidated. Oxytalan fibers, which adhere to tropoelastin in the lowest degree, are completely missing in photoaged dermis. The decomposition of elastic fibers is due to the action of neprilysin, a member of the serine metalloproteinase family [57], and neutrophil elastase, a member of the serine proteinase family [58]. Neprilysin activity in dermal fibroblasts is increased by UVA or IL-1α [59]. The infiltration of neutrophils into the dermis is stimulated by CXCL8/IL-8, which is secreted from keratinocytes following exposure to UVB irradiation or high oxidation conditions [60].

3.5.2 The Anti-Aging Effects of Phytochemicals

UVB-irradiated keratinocytes secrete inflammatory cytokines such as IL-18/IL-8, which is sethat up-regulates and activates MMP-1 in fibroblasts. Therefore, to suppress ROS production in keratinocytes is an attractive strategy for improving dermal conditions. Passion fruit (*Passiflora edulis* Sims.) has a strong anti-oxidant ability since it contains multiple polyphenolic compounds. Although the CM from UVB-irradiated keratinocytes induces the activation of MMP-1 in fibroblasts, the CM from UVB-irradiated keratinocytes in the presence of passion fruit significantly suppresses MMP-1 activity [61].

3.5.3 Assay Protocols for UVA-Induced Alterations of Dermal Remodeling

3.5.3.1 Type I collagen determination by ELISA

Fibroblasts secrete type I collagen peptides into the culture medium. Thus, collagen synthesis by fibroblasts can be determined by quantifying the amount of type I collagen peptide in the culture medium using an ELISA.

3.5.3.2 Formation of collagen fibers visualized by immunostaining

Fibroblasts build collagen fibers during culture for 1 week or 2 weeks. The dishes with cultured fibroblasts are fixed with 4% formaldehyde and then immunostained with an anti-collagen type I antibody. Nuclei are stained with Hoechst 33342. Fluorescence images are observed using a fluorescence microscope [62].

3.5.3.3 Western blotting of MMP-1

Fibroblasts secrete MMP-1 into the culture medium and that MMP-1 can be detected by western blot analysis of the culture medium.

3.6 CONCLUSION

The authors have introduced the concepts of the skin care efficacies of phytochemicals based on the causative mechanisms and factors that disrupt skin health and skin beauty, and discussed the methods used to assess those processes and the products formulated. In addition, to assist understanding, we introduced studies that evaluated phytochemicals as case studies.

The authors hope that this chapter helps in the design of suitable assessment methods for studies of phytochemicals.

REFERENCES

1. Herrling Th, Jung K, Fuchs J. Measurements of UV-generated free radicals/reactive oxygen species (ROS) in skin. Spectrochim Acta A Mol Biomol Spectrosc. 2006;63(4):840–5.
2. Gonzalez Maglio DH, Paz ML, Ferrari A, et al. Skin damage and mitochondrial dysfunction after acute ultraviolet B irradiation: relationship with nitric oxide production. Photodermatol Photoimmunol Photomed. 2005;21(6):311–7.
3. Beak SM, Lee YS, Kim JA. NADPH oxidase and cyclooxygenase mediate the ultraviolet B-induced generation of reactive oxygen species and activation of nuclear factor-κB in HaCaT human keratinocytes. Biochimie. 2004;86(7):425–9.
4. Mizutani T, Sumida H, Sagawa Y, et al. Carbonylated proteins exposed to UVA and to blue light generate reactive oxygen species through a type I photosensitizing reaction. J Dermatol Sci. 2016;84(3):314–21.
5. Maeda H, Akaike T. Nitric oxide and oxygen radicals in infection, inflammation, and cancer. Biochemistry. 1998;63(7):854–65.
6. Lee JM, Johnson JA. An important role of Nrf2-ARE pathway in the cellular defense mechanism. J Biochem Mol Biol. 2004;37(2):139–43.
7. Toyama T, Wada-Takahashi S, Takamichi M, et al. Reactive oxygen species scavenging activity of *Jixueteng* evaluated by electron spin resonance (ESR) and photon emission. Nat Prod Commun. 2014;9(12):1755–9.
8. Mizutani T, Masaki H. Anti-photoaging capability of antioxidant extract from *Camellia japonica* leaf. Exp Dermatol. 2014;23(Suppl 1):23–6.
9. Oh Y, Lim HW, Huang YH, et al. Attenuating properties of *Agastache rugosa* leaf extract against ultraviolet-B-induced photoaging via up-regulating glutathione and superoxide dismutase in a human keratinocyte cell line. J Photochem Photobiol B. 2016;163:170–6.
10. Schadich E, Hlaváč J, Volná T, et al. Effects of ginger phenylpropanoids and quercetin on Nrf2-ARE pathway in human BJ fibroblasts and HaCaT keratinocytes. Biomed Res Int. 2016;2016:2173275.
11. Masaki H, Atsumi T, Sakurai H. Hamamelitannin as a new potent active oxygen scavenger. Phytochemistry. 1994;37(2):337–43.
12. Ogiwara T, Satoh K, Kadoma Y, et al. Radical scavenging activity and cytotoxicity of ferulic acid. Anticancer Res. 2002;22(5):2711–7.
13. Katsuyama Y, Tsuboi T, Taira N, et al. 3-*O*-Laurylglyceryl ascorbate activates the intracellular antioxidant system through the contribution of PPAR-γ and Nrf2. J Dermatol Sci. 2016;82(3):189–96.
14. Yamawaki Y, Mizutani T, Okano Y, et al. The impact of carbonylated proteins on the skin and potential agents to block their effects. Exp Dermatol. 2019;28(Suppl 1):32–7.
15. Masaki H, Yamashita Y, Kyotani D, et al. Correlations between skin hydration parameters and corneocyte-derived parameters to characterize skin conditions. J Cosmet Dermatol. 2019;18(1):308–14.
16. Endo K, Mizutani T, Okano Y, et al. A red pumpkin seed extract reduces melanosome transfer to keratinocytes by activation of Nrf2 signaling. J Cosmet Dermatol. 2019;18(3):827–34.

17. Katsuyama Y, Taira N, Tsuboi T, et al. 3-*O*-Laurylglyceryl ascorbate reinforces skin barrier function through not only the reduction of oxidative stress but also the activation of ceramide synthesis. Int J Cosmet Sci. 2017;39(1):49–55.

18. Mizutani T, Yamawaki Y, Okano Y, et al. Oxidative stress initiated by the depletion of endogenous antioxidants induces dysfunction of the epidermal barrier. The 30th IFSCC Munich Congress: Proceedings. 2018.

19. Kikuchi K, Kobayashi H, Hirao T, et al. Improvement of mild inflammatory changes of the facial skin induced by winter environment with daily applications of a moisturizing cream. A half-side test of biophysical skin parameters, cytokine expression pattern and the formation of cornified envelope. Dermatology. 2003;207(3):269–75.

20. Kobayashi Y, Iwai I, Akutsu N, et al. Increased carbonyl protein levels in the stratum corneum of the face during winter. Int J Cosmet Sci. 2008;30(1):35–40.

21. Yokota M, Shimizu K, Kyotani D, et al. The possible involvement of skin dryness on alterations of the dermal matrix. Exp Dermatol. 2014;23(Suppl 1):27–31.

22. Ishikawa J, Shimotoyodome Y, Chen S, et al. Eucalyptus increases ceramide levels in keratinocytes and improves stratum corneum function. Int J Cosmet Sci. 2012;34(1):17–22.

23. Ishikawa J, Yoshida H, Ito S, et al. Dry skin in the winter is related to the ceramide profile in the stratum corneum and can be improved by treatment with a Eucalyptus extract. J Cosmet Dermatol. 2013;12(1):3–11.

24. Matts PJ, Oblong JE, Bissett DL. A review of the range of effects of niacinamide in human skin. IFSCC Magazine. 2002;5(4):285–9.

25. Bierman JC, Laughlin T, Tamura M, et al. Niacinamide mitigates SASP-related inflammation induced by environmental stressors in human epidermal keratinocytes and skin. Int J Cosmet Sci. 2020;42(5):501–11.

26. Harding CR, Aho S, Bosko CA. Filaggrin – revisited. Int J Cosmet Sci. 2013;35(5):412–23.

27. Michel S, Schmidt R, Shroot B, et al. Morphological and biochemical characterization of the cornified envelopes from human epidermal keratinocytes of different origin. J Invest Dermatol. 1988;91(1):11–5.

28. Elias PM, Gruber R, Crumrine D, et al. Formation and functions of the corneocyte lipid envelope (CLE). Biochim Biophys Acta. 2014;1841(3):314–8.

29. Eckert RL, Sturniolo MT, Broome AM, et al. Transglutaminase function in epidermis. J Invest Dermatol. 2005;124(3):481–92.

30. Behne M, Uchida Y, Seki T, et al. Omega-hydroxyceramides are required for corneocyte lipid envelope (CLE) formation and normal epidermal permeability barrier function. J Invest Dermatol. 2000;114(1):185–92.

31. Coderch L, López O, Maza A, et al. Ceramides and skin function. Am J Clin Dermatol. 2003;4(2):107–29.

32. Hanada K. Serine palmitoyltransferase, a key enzyme of sphingolipid metabolism. Biochim Biophys Acta. 2003;1632(1–3):16–30.

33. Schneeberger EE, Lynch RD. The tight junction: a multifunctional complex. Am J Physiol Cell Physiol. 2004;286(6):C1213–28.

34. Hirao T, Denda M, Takahashi M. Identification of immature cornified envelopes in the barrier-impaired epidermis by characterization of their hydrophobicity and antigenicities of the components. Exp Dermatol. 2001;10(1):35–44.

35. Goorochurn R, Viennet C, Granger C, et al. Biological processes in solar lentigo: insights brought by experimental models. Exp Dermatol. 2016;25(3):174–7.

36. Cario-Andre M, Lepreux S, Pain C, et al. Perilesional vs. lesional skin changes in senile lentigo. J Cutan Pathol. 2004;31(6):441–7.

37. Iriyama S, Ono T, Aoki H, et al. Hyperpigmentation in human solar lentigo is promoted by heparanase-induced loss of heparan sulfate chains at the dermal–epidermal junction. J Dermatol Sci. 2011;64(3):223–8.

38. Yoon JE, Kim Y, Kwon S, et al. Senescent fibroblasts drive ageing pigmentation: a potential therapeutic target for senile lentigo. Theranostics. 2018;8(17):4620–32.

39. Hirobe T. Keratinocytes regulate the function of melanocytes. Dermatol Sin. 2014;32(4):200–4.

40. Cario-André M, Pain C, Gauthier Y, et al. *In vivo* and *in vitro* evidence of dermal fibroblasts influence on human epidermal pigmentation. Pigment Cell Res. 2006;19(5):434–42.

41. Beak SM, Lee YS, Kim JA, et al. NADPH oxidase and cyclooxygenase mediate the ultraviolet Binduced generation of reactive oxygen species and activation of nuclear factor-kappaB in HaCaT human keratinocytes, Biochimie. 2004;86(7):425–9.

42. Hachiya A, Kobayashi A, Yoshida Y, et al. Biphasic expression of two paracrine melanogenic cytokines, stem cell factor and endothelin-1, in ultraviolet B-induced human melanogenesis. Am J Pathol. 2004;165(6):2099–109.

43. Bolognia J, Murray M, Pawelek J. UVB-induced melanogenesis may be mediated through the MSH-receptor system. J Invest Dermatol. 1989;92(5):651–6.

44. Tomita Y, Iwamoto M, Masuda T, et al. Stimulatory effect of prostaglandin E2 on the configuration of normal human melanocytes *in vitro*. J Invest Dermatol. 1987;89(3):299–301.

45. Ando H, Niki Y, Ito M, et al. Melanosomes are transferred from melanocytes to keratinocytes through the processes of packaging, release, uptake, and dispersion. J Invest Dermatol. 2012;132(4):1222–9.

46. Jung E, Lee JA, Shin S, et al. Madecassoside inhibits melanin synthesis by blocking ultraviolet-induced inflammation. Molecules. 2013;18(12):15724–36.

47. Ochiai Y, Kaburagi S, Obayashi K, et al. A new lipophilic pro-vitamin C, tetra-isopalmitoyl ascorbic acid (VC-IP), prevents UV-induced skin pigmentation through its anti-oxidative properties. J Dermatol Sci. 2006;44(1):37–44.

48. Amano S. Possible involvement of basement membrane damage in skin photoaging. J Invest Dermatol Symp Proc. 2009;14(1):2–7.

49. Kligman LH, Akin FJ, Kligman AM. The contributions of UVA and UVB to connective tissue damage in hairless mice. J Invest Dermatol. 1985;84(4):272–6.

50. Naylor EC, Watson REB, Sherratt MJ. Molecular aspects of skin ageing. Maturitas. 2011;69(3):249–56.

51. Nishimori Y, Edwards C, Pearse A, et al. Degenerative alterations of dermal collagen fiber bundles in photodamaged human skin and UV-irradiated hairless mouse skin: possible effect on decreasing skin mechanical properties and appearance of wrinkles. J Invest Dermatol. 2001;117(6):1458–63.

52. Papageorgis P, Stylianopoulos T. Role of TGFβ in regulation of the tumor microenvironment and drug delivery. Int J Oncol. 2015;46(3):933–43.

53. Fligiel SEG, Varani J, Datta SC, et al. Collagen degradation in aged/photodamaged skin *in vivo* and after exposure to matrix metalloproteinase-1 in vitro. J Invest Dermatol. 2003;120(5):842–8.

54. Gupta A, Rosenberger SF, Bowden GT. Increased ROS levels contribute to elevated transcription factor and MAP kinase activities in malignantly progressed mouse keratinocyte cell lines. Carcinogenesis. 1999;20(11):2063–73.

55. Peus D, Vasa RA, Beyerle A, et al. UVB activates ERK1/2 and p38 signaling pathways via reactive oxygen species in cultured keratinocytes. J Invest Dermatol. 1999;112(5):751–6.

56. Wagenseil JE, Mecham RP. New insights into elastic fiber assembly. Birth Defects Res C Embryo Today. 2007;81(4):229–40.

57. Huertas ACM, Schmelzer CEH, Luise C, et al. Degradation of tropoelastin and skin elastin by neprilysin. Biochimie. 2018;146:73–8.

58. F Rijken, Bruijnzeel PLB. The pathogenesis of photoaging: the role of neutrophils and neutrophil-derived enzymes. J Invest Dermatol Symp Proc. 2009;14(1):67–72.

59. Morisaki N, Moriwaki S, Sugiyama-Nakagiri Y, et al. Neprilysin is identical to skin fibroblast elastase. J Biol Chem. 2010;285(51):39819–27.

60. Strickland I, Rhodes LE, Flanagan BF, et al. TNF-alpha and IL-8 are upregulated in the epidermis of normal human skin after UVB exposure: correlation with neutrophil accumulation and E-selectin expression. J Invest Dermatol. 1997;108(5):763–8.

61. Maruki-Uchida H, Kurita I, Sugiyama K, et al. The protective effects of piceatannol from passion fruit (*Passiflora edulis*) seeds in UVB-irradiated keratinocytes. Biol Pharm Bull. 2013;36(5):845–9.

62. Pajorova J, Bacakova M, Musilkova J, et al. Morphology of a fibrin nanocoating influences dermal fibroblast behavior. Int J Nanomed. 2018;13:3367–80.

4

Phytocosmetics for Skin Care

Mayuree Kanlayavattanakul and Nattaya Lourith

Contents

4.1 INTRODUCTION

The aesthetic benefits of natural-derived actives – especially those of phytocosmetics – have dramatically increased in demand among consumers. Consumers' preferences are supported with the scientific evidence from researchers. Complementary and alternative medicines from available plants in traditional medicines have been explored for their cutaneous benefits, in addition to any other beneficial effects. This chapter is devoted to the phytocosmetic actives claimed to have good chemical and biological profiles for skin aging, skin lightening, acne, greasy skin, and skin dryness. The causes of each skin disorders are briefly addressed in order to outline appropriate solutions. Thereafter, phytocosmetics for skin aging, lightening, dryness, acne and greasy treatments are summarized alphabetically on the basis of their pharmacologically actives and evidence for efficacy in human volunteers.

4.2 PHYTOCOSMETICS FOR SKIN AGING TREATMENT

Skin aging is caused by several factors, mainly oxidants or radicals damaging/accumulating/exacerbating damage to cell membranes and components, resulting in aging of skin [1, 2].

Degradation of cutaneous cellular collagen and elastin fibers including glycosaminoglycans (GAGs); hyaluronan, chondroitin, keratin, dermatan, and heparin or so called extracellular matrix (ECM) reverses skin elasticity and tensile strength. The matrix metalloproteinases (MMPs; MMP-1 to MMP-28) are the degradation enzymes whose function is accelerated with age, accumulating with radicals, including inflammatory mediators. In addition to basic screening of anti-oxidant activity, inhibitory effects against the relevant enzymes and inflammatory mediators including the capability promoting/retaining ECM production are thus the key strategies for determining the potential of an active prior to examination *in vivo*. In this respect, consumers are most familiar with the commercialized anti-aging products containing anti-oxidants [1, 2].

Phytocosmetic actives with the supportive evidence for safety and efficacy in human volunteers have been conclusively summarized for the treatment of skin aging. The preparation, standardization and biological evaluations are outside the scope of this chapter as regards *in vivo* non-invasive methods for cutaneous aging evaluations. Readers will find this elsewhere [1, 2] and in different chapters of this book.

4.2.1 Anethum graveolens

Dill seed extract, the lysyl oxidase-like enzyme (an extracellular enzyme catalyzing the cross-linking between microfibrils, and tropoelastin expression in dermal fibroblasts, promoter), is one of the phytocosmetic actives combating aging commercially produced by several cosmetic suppliers (BASF, etc.). The active emulsion was extract (1%) has clinically proven anti-aging activity. The active emulsion was applied onto the face of 50 female volunteers (43–56 years old) two times a day for 3 months consecutively. Skin elasticity was significantly (p = 0.035) improved after 56 days of treatment; facial aging appeared notably (p = 0.02) improved at the end of the observation period (84 days). Anti-aging efficacy was confirmed with facial wrinkle reduction in terms of wrinkle length and area (p = 0.002 and 0.011) [3].

4.2.2 Arctium lappa

Burdock's fruit contains the anti-aging active arctiin. Arctiin possesses cellular anti-inflammatory effect, from tumor necrosis factor-alpha (TNF-α) and interleukin-6 (IL-6) with MMP-1 suppression and stimulation activity on collagen synthesis in fibroblasts. The formulation containing burdock fruit extract (1.2%, 0.25% arctiin) significantly increased the pro-collagen level ($p = 0.0103$), hyaluronan synthase-2 expression ($p = 0.0184$), and hyaluronan content, as clinically evaluated on the inner forearms of 40 females (39–65 years old) for 12 weeks (two times a day). Facial aging treatment with this phytocosmetic showed significant ($p = 0.05$) crow's feet wrinkle area reduction with the product for 4 weeks by volunteer treated with the same group of volunteer treated with the product for 4 weeks by the same application [4].

4.2.3 Areca catechu

Betel nut has been shown to inhibit in vitro elastase and hyaluronidase activities [5]. In addition, the extract showed cellular activity against human leukocyte elastase at IC_{50} 48.1 µg/ml, with a significant ($p < 0.05$) proliferation stimulating human fibroblasts (85%) and collagen synthesis (40%) at a dilution of 10^{-4}% compared with ascorbic acid. The extract cream (3%) was clinically assessed in 20 volunteers following twice daily topical application for 6 weeks. Skin elasticity was significantly improved ($p < 0.05$, 35%), with significant reduction of roughness ($p < 0.05$, 16.7%) and wrinkle depth (23%) [6].

4.2.4 Aspalathus linearis

Red tea or rooibos with anti-oxidant flavonoids has cutaneous benefits, driving its commercially available extract for the cosmetic industry (Tealine®, Cosmetochem, etc.). Red tea gel (0.15%) showed a remarkable wrinkle reduction (9.9%) over the control following a twice daily application for 28 days by 20 female volunteers [7].

4.2.5 Camellia sinensis

Tea is regarded as a rich source of health benefits catechins that are also appreciable for aging treatment [7]. Green tea cream (86% catechins) diminished the accumulating effect of photoaging by suppressing oxidative stress and inflammation as explored in animal models [8, 9]. Along with its anti-inflammatory ability, DNA damage in human skin was reduced after the application of epi-gallocatechin gallate (10%) three times a week for 6 weeks in 11 male volunteers from 5% green tea extract [10, 11].

4.2.6 Centella asiatica

C. asiatica is traditionally used for photoaging protection [12]. Its anti-aging ability is contributed by madescassoside, asiaticoside, centelloside, and asiatic acid that enhance collagen production *via* a collagen stimulating effect in dermal fibroblasts. Skin care products containing 0.1% madescassoside isolated from *C. asiatica* significantly (p < 0.0001) increased skin elasticity as demonstrated in 20 female volunteers (45–60 years old) who applied the product two times a day for 6 months [13].

4.2.7 Gingko biloba

Gingko is well-known as a longevity remedy with regard to its anti-oxidaive phenolics and flavonoids, especially ginkolides and bilobalide. Gingko phytochemical cosmetic active extract is therefore widely commercialized for the cosmetics industry (e.g. Flavonids complex SC®, Cosmetochem). Gingko has evidence for efficacy in the commercial available anti-wrinkle ginkgo cosmetics [7].

4.2.8 Litchi chinensis

Skin elasticity and wrinkle reduction was significantly (p < 0.05 and p < 0.005) achieved by 0.1% litchi serum. The efficacy of litchi serums was confirmed by a split-face, randomized, single-blind controlled study showing that a 0.1% litchi serum was significantly (p < 0.05) better than a 0.05% version [14].

4.2.9 Nelumbo nucifera

Lotus extract has potent anti-radical activity with an inhibitory effect against elastase. The extract (1%) was shown to be non-skin irritating in 20 volunteers using patch testing for 24 h [15]. Anti-aging efficacy on facial skin was exhibited in 11 male volunteers applying a multiple emulsion containing the extract (2.5%) once a day for 8 weeks. Skin roughness was significantly improved (2.5%, 18.10%), skin wrinkling (p = 0.032, 18.10%), skin wrinkling (p = 0.045, 10.92%), skin wrinkling (p = 0.048, 11.22%), and skin smoothness (p = 0.003, 19.33%) [16].

4.2.10 *Oryza sativa*

Jasmine rice panicle extract was shown to have a high content of *p*-coumaric, ferulic, and caffeic acids [17], and was not cytotoxic to cutaneous cell lines [18]. Anti-aging efficacy of the jasmine rice panicle preparations (0.1–0.2%) was confirmed by their potency for skin firmness and smoothness, in addition to a reduction in skin wrinkling as evidenced in the clinical trial in 24 volunteers over 84 days of treatment [18].

4.2.11 *Paeonia lactiflora*

Peony extract containing more than 60% of paeoniflorin showed cellular anti-inflammatory activities and a protective effect against UVB-induced DNA damage in human keratinocytes. The anti-wrinkle cream (0.5% paeoniflorin) was twice daily applied onto the face by 20 female volunteers for 8 weeks; surface roughness of facial skin was significantly improved ($p < 0.05$, 17.65%) [19].

4.2.12 *Sanguisorba officinalis*

This oriental medicinal plant (Ji-Yu in Korean) was demonstrated *in vitro* and *ex vivo* as an anti-oxidant with inhibition and suppression of elastase and MMP-1 activities including collagen type I synthesis promotion. The active compound is ziyuglycoside I. Anti-wrinkle cream (0.03% ziyuglycoside I) significantly ($p < 0.05$) reduced skin roughness as examined in 20 female volunteers for 12 weeks [20].

4.2.13 *Silybum marianum*

Milk thistle containing silymarin as the main component, with anti-oxidant and anti-inflammatory activities, has been used for photoaging protection [21]. The anti-aging efficacy of milk thistle (4%) cream was confirmed in 11 male volunteers after 12 weeks treatment with a reduction of skin roughness, scaliness, and wrinkles [22].

4.2.14 *Uttwiler spatlauber*

Swiss apple, with a cellular healing activity in H_2O_2-damaged fibroblasts, has efficacy claimed for its anti-wrinkle activity, and is current commercialized

(PhytoCellTech™ Malus Domestica, Mibelle Biochemistry). Volunteers [20] treated with 2% of active cream were documented with a reduction of crow's feet area and facial wrinkles [23].

4.2.15 *Zanthoxylum bungeanum*

Szechuan pepper is one of a number of important phytocosmetic sources patented for cutaneous applications including for aging treatment as a skin-soothing agent (Zanthalene®, Indena S.A.S.). Cosmetics containing the commercialized extract (1% and 2%) were clinically evaluated in 21 female volunteers (35–65 years old) for 4 weeks of application (twice daily); facial skin lifting efficacy was revealed [24].

4.3 PHYTOCOSMETICS FOR SKIN LIGHTENING

Hyperpigmentation of skin, skin dullness, and darkening skin are accumulated by several factors, chiefly radicals and inflammatory mediators [2]. Briefly, keratinocytes are UV stimulated secreting α-melanocyte stimulating hormone (α-MSH) that further bind to melanocortin 1 receptors (MC1R) expressed on the surface of melanocytes, inducing melanogenesis via multiple signaling pathways resulting from cAMP, protein kinase A (PKA), cAMP response element-binding protein (CREB), and microphthalmia-associated transcription factor (MITF) activity. MITF transcribe melanogenic enzymes, i.e. tyrosinase, tyrosinase-related protein (TRP)-1 and TRP-2. In a different pathway, melanogenesis is controlled by mitogen-activated protein kinases (MAPKs) controlling melanogenesis. MAPKs are modulated by nuclear factor E2-related factor 2 (Nrf2). These are stimulated by cytokines, oxidative stress, radical, and UV.

Phytocosmetics for skin lightening agents that are certified safe and efficiently used in cosmetic products are summarized next.

4.3.1 *Cassia fistula*

The extract of golden shower tree pods with *in vitro* tyrosinase inhibitory effect was proven to have skin lightening efficacy. An emulsion (5%) efficiently brightens the facial skin of 17 volunteers who applied the preparation twice daily for 12 consecutive weeks. A remarkable skin lightening (p < 0.0001) was observed following the first week treatment (7.0%), with clear improvements evident at the end of the study (13.0%) [25].

4.3.2 *Glycyrrhiza glabra*

Licorice is a plant well known for treatment of skin dullness with glabridin. Glabridin is a stronger mushroom tyrosinase inhibitor than kojic acid [26]. Along with its anti-melanogenesis activity in B16 melanoma cells and guinea pig [27], licorice extract containing glabridin has confirmed skin lightening efficacy in reducing dark spots on skin in human volunteers [28].

4.3.3 *Hippophae rhamnoides*

An emulsion containing 5% of the *in vitro* sea buckthorn extract was shown to have efficacy in skin melanin content reduction in 19 volunteers who applied twice daily the emulsion facially for 12 weeks. Facial melanin content reduction was noted at the first week (3.5%) of application; skin lightening efficacy was increased and significantly improved (16.35%, p < 0.0001) by the end of the study [25].

4.3.4 *Litchi chinensis*

The efficacy of litchi serums was confirmed by a split-face, randomized, single-blind controlled study showing that the 0.1% litchi serum was significantly (p < 0.05) better than the 0.05% one. Skin lightening efficacy of the 0.1% and 0.05% litchi serum was significantly (p < 0.001 and p < 0.05) higher than the placebo [14].

4.3.5 *Oenothera biennis*

The saponified oil of evening primrose (12.5 µg/ml) significantly suppressed melanogenesis in B16F10 melanoma cells. The oil is highly safe as the non-toxic dose was high (100 µg/ml), which pronouncedly suppressed melanin production (12.8 ± 1.8%). Anti-melanogenesis was governed by its fatty acid components linoleic acid (65–75%), linolenic acid (7–10%) and oleic acid (9%). The mechanism was shown to work by suppressing messenger RNA (mRNA) expression of TRP-1, TRP-2, and MITF. Thereafter, UVB-induced hyperpigmentation forearm skin was efficiently treated by a twice daily application of the oil for 2 months; a significant improvement was measurable after 1 month of treatment. However, the clinical study was examined in a small group of the volunteers, 3 men [29].

4.3.6 *Oryza sativa*

Rice phenolics such as *p*-coumaric acid, caffeic acid, ferulic acid, and gallic acid are of importance in skin remedies [17]. Rice panicles enriched with these phenolics inhibited mushroom tyrosinase and suppressed melanogenesis in B16F10 melanoma cells via tyrosinase and TRP-2 inhibitory effects. Rice panicle extract (0.1% and 0.2%) creams were shown to have skin lightening efficacy that significantly ($p < 0.001$) improved after 28 days and was more pronounced by the end of the study (84 days) following a twice daily application in 24 volunteers [18].

4.3.7 *Punica granatum*

Phenolic-rich pomegranate peel extract exhibited strong anti-oxidant activity with an *in vitro* tyrosinase inhibitory effect. Its potency for treating skin hyperpigmentation was confirmed by the suppression of cellular melanogenesis through tyrosinase and TRP-2 inhibitions as examined in the B16F10 melanoma cells. The extract was developed into a stable serum and mask. The products were demonstrated to be non-irritating in 30 Thai volunteers participating in a single application closed patch test. A split-face, randomized, double-blind, placebo-controlled test of the skin lightening effect was evaluated in the volunteers over 28 consecutive daily treatments. The active serum and mask were better in facial skin lightening efficacy than the placebo ($p < 0.005$) [30].

4.3.8 *Zea may*

Corn bran rich in hydroxycinnamic acids suppressed melanin synthesis in B16F1 melanoma cells via MITF suppression. Skin lightening efficacy was assessed in 21 female volunteers whose back was tanned by UV irradiation, with topical application of the corn bran (0.1%) cream two times a day for 8 consecutive weeks. Skin lightening efficacy was significantly improved after 4 weeks (11%) and more progress with time (15% after 6 weeks and 19% after 8 weeks) [31].

4.4 PHYTOCOSMETICS FOR DRIED SKIN TREATMENT

Phyto-actives polysaccharides are especially promising skin hydrating agents. They create hydrogel or hydrocolloid gel structures, mobilizing water to the contacted skin [32, 33]. Phytocosmetic botanical polysaccharides are therefore summarized in this section.

4.4.1 *Abelmoschus esculentus*

Okra is an important source of polysaccharide with high content of the fruit mucilage. Moisturizing alcohol-based hand rub containing okra polysaccharide has been formulated. This moisturizing product with 0.105% polysaccharide maintained skin hydration significantly better than the placebo in 20 volunteers [34].

4.4.2 *Aloe vera*

The leaf enriched with polysaccharides is widely used in skin preparation and popularly sold over-the-counter (OTC) for its skin nourishing effect. Aloe polysaccharide in a topical product (0.1%, 0.25%, and 0.5%) significantly increased skin hydration as examined in 20 volunteers monitored after 1 and 2 weeks of application [35].

4.4.3 *Basella alba*

Ceylon spinach polysaccharide extract (0.05–0.10%) 7–28% hydrated skin as evaluated in 22 volunteers throughout the observation time (0–210 min) following a single application [36].

4.4.4 *Dendrobium*

White orchid (*Dendrobium* cv. Khao Sanan) polysaccharide with antioxidant activity was demonstrated to have skin hydrating efficacy in 22 Thai volunteers [37].

4.4.5 *Durio zebethinus*

Durian is enriched with polysaccharides in the hull. The polysaccharide was formulated into gel (10%) and assessed on its skin hydrating activity in 18 volunteers for 8 weeks twice daily (morning and evening). Skin water content was significantly increased at the first examination following treatment of 4 weeks (p = 0.024) and improved (p = 0.003) at the end of the study. The results additionally revealed that the efficacy in female volunteers was better than in male. In addition, the product imparted excellent enhancement of skin hydration in the subjects younger than 30 years old, a better result than for those who were older [38].

4.4.6 *Malva sylvestris (Scaphium scaphigerum)*

Malva nut is widely applied for dermatological therapeutic effects. The herb's potential in skin hydration is governed by its abundant mucilage. Malva mucilage was formulated into skin hydration products. The skin hydrating efficacy was shown to exhibit improved performance over benchmark tamarind and algae polysaccharide gels (after 180 min observation) as assessed in 24 volunteers [39].

4.4.7 *Piptadenia colubrina*

This leguminous tree of the South American rain forest had skin beneficial polysaccharide isolated with the extractive yield of 0.05–0.25%. The extracted polysaccharide was further formulated into a gel-cream product (5%). Skin capacitance was significantly improved in 15 volunteers after 14 days treatment [40].

4.4.8 *Ulmus davidiana*

The root of *U. davidiana* var. *japonica*, used traditionally in Oriental medicine, was examined for its benefits for skin. The polysaccharide derived from the plant root with a molecular weight of 20 KDa, consisting mainly of rhamnose (57.37%), was shown first for water retaining *in vitro*, including its safety and activity in human skin fibroblasts. Established as a non-cytotoxic polysaccharide with water holding capacity, it additionally suppressed inflammatory mediators as evidenced by the reduction of PEG_2, IL-6, and IL-8 in the cultured cells. Moisturizing activity of the polysaccharide was further assessed in 10 female volunteers. The skin hydrating effect was almost the same as the HA used as the positive control [41].

4.5 PHYTOCOSMETICS FOR ACNE AND GREASY SKIN TREATMENTS

Acne is regulated by sebum hypersecretion in deformed follicles, which leads to microcomedones and the follicular hyperproliferation of microcomedones, causing inflammation and comedones in both open and closed types (black and white comedones) appearing in papules, pustules, nodules, and cysts. The resulting skin condition with sebum enrichment is prone to the anaerobic growth of *Propionibacterium acnes*, the main causative microorganism in acne. In addition, *Staphylococcus epidermidis* and *Pitryosporum ovale* are present in acne lesions. Proliferation of these microorganisms, mainly *P. acnes*, leads to inflammatory lesions and severe acne. Skin inflammation is initiated by CD4+ in T lymphocytes, regulated by toll-like receptors (TLRs) following neutrophil infiltration, generating reactive oxygen species and protease enzymes, leading to follicular wall rupture of sebaceous glands. This changes the composition of sebum; in particular, linoleic acid and hyperkeratinization are initiated as well as a reduction in desquamation. Subsequently, the proinflammatory cytokines, nuclear factor κB (NF-κB), IL, TNF, interferon (IFN), lipopolysachharide (LPS), transforming growth factor (TGF), prostaglandin (PG), and gamma and granulocyte-macrophage colony-stimulating factor (GM-CSF) are released, causing microcomedones. The resulting microcomedones further develop into comedones and inflammatory lesions [42].

4.5.1 *Camelia sinensis*

A facial tonner containing green tea has been developed and its anti-greasy properties evaluated in 20 volunteers. Green tea toners (2%, 4.5%, and 7%) had efficacy of 3.47 ± 0.10, 8.18 ± 0.44, and $17.87 \pm 0.46\%$ following 14 days of facial treatment. The efficiency was more pronounced at the end of the study; day 28 (8.48 ± 0.13, 20.26 ± 1.03, and $31.57 \pm 1.22\%$). Anti-sebum efficacy of the 4.5 and 7% green tea toners were significantly better than the base formula (day 14; p < 0.05, day 28; p < 0.01). The efficacy at 28 days treatment was significantly better than 14 days (p < 0.05) [43].

4.5.2 *Melaleuca alternifolia*

Tea tree oil has been regarded as an efficient phytocosmetic active for acne treatment on the basis of inhibitory effects against *S. aureus, S. epidermidis*, and *P. acnes* of its major components, terpinen-4-ol, α-terpineol, and α-pinene [44]. Tea tree oil gel effectively reduced acne lesions comparable with benzoyl peroxide at the same concentration with fewer side effects [45]. Therefore, it is one of the most popular and effective OTC acne treatments.

4.5.3 *Psidium guajava*

Guava was developed into facial toners. The 6% guava extract toner significantly reduced oiliness of forehead (13.10 ± 3.67%, p < 0.05) and nose (21.43 ± 3.21%, p < 0.001) better than the base toner. Its activity on the nose was significantly noted (10.72 ± 3.51%, p < 0.05) from the third week of application [46].

4.6 CONCLUSION

Skin beneficial plants are summarized in Table 4.1. It should be noted that several cosmetic benefits can be claimed for one plant. In addition, phytocosmetic ingredients in the forms of isolated pure compounds and extracts (i.e. selected active principles and oil) have been popularly incorporated in the commercialized skin care preparations listed from the top best-selling products retrieved from Amazon (see Table 4.1). It should be noted that there might be something of a gap between the scientific evidence-based plants and the commercialized ones. The cosmetic scientists are therefore encouraged to bridge these gaps in order to maximize the usage of phytocosmetics fulfilling consumer expectations of the safety and efficacy of phytocosmetics.

TABLE 4.1 Phytocosmetics for skin care

NAME		BENEFITS			
SCIENTIFIC	COMMON	AGING	LIGHTENING	DRYNESS	ACNE AND GREASY
Abelmoschus esculentus	Okra			✓	
Aloe vera	Aloe			✓	
Anethum graveolens	Dill	✓			
Arctium lappa	Burdock	✓			
Areca catechu	Betel	✓			
Aspalathus linearis	Rooibos	✓			
Basella alba	Ceylon spinach			✓	
Camellia sinensis	Tea	✓			✓
Cassia fistula	Golden shower tree		✓		
Centella asiatica	Asiatic pennywort	✓			
Dendrobium spp.	Orchid			✓	
Durio zebethinus	Durian			✓	
Gingko biloba	Gingko	✓			
Glycyrrhiza glabra	Licorice		✓		
Hippophae rhamnoides	Sea buckthorn		✓		
Litchi chinensis	Litchi	✓	✓		
Malva sylvestris	Mallow			✓	
Melaleuca alternifolia	Tea tree				✓
Nelumbo nucifera	Lotus	✓			
Oenothera biennis	Evening primrose		✓		
Oryza sativa	Rice	✓	✓		
Paeonia lactiflora	Peony	✓			
Psidium guajava	Guava				✓

TABLE 4.1 (Continued)

		AGING	LIGHTENING	DRYNESS	ACNE AND GREASY
NAME		BENEFITS			
SCIENTIFIC	COMMON	AGING	LIGHTENING	DRYNESS	ACNE AND GREASY
Piptadenia colubrina	Angico-branco			✓	
Punica granatum	Pomegranate		✓		
Sanguisorba officinalis	Great burnet	✓			
Silybum marianum	Milk thistle	✓			
Ulmus davidiana	Japanese elm			✓	
Uttwiler spatlauber	Swiss apple	✓			
Zanthoxylum bungeanum	Szechuan pepper	✓			
Zea may	Corn	✓			

Phytocosmetic ingredients

EXTRACT	ACTIVE
Almond, almond oil, aloe, apple stem cells, apricot, avocado oil, blueberry, burdock, borage seed oil, calendula oil, *Calendula officinalis*, *Calophylum inophylum* oil, *Centella asiatica*, chamomile, cocoa butter, coconut, coconut oil, cucumber, *Cyathea medullaris*, dill, *Eclipta alba*, evening primrose oil, *Fagus sylvatica*, ginseng, goji, grape stem cells, grape seed, grape seed oil, guar, mulberry, *Helichrysum italicum*, *Hibicus sabdariffa*, horsetail, hop, juniper oil, jojoba oil, lavender, lavender oil, *Lilium candidum*, *Limonium vulgare*, linseed, *Lonicera caprifolium*, lotus, macadamia oil, malva nut, marigold, moringa oil, oat, olive, olive oil, onion, *Onopordum acanthium*, orange oil, patchouli oil, *Plantago major*, *Pelargonium graveolens* oil, *Pfaffia paniculata*, *Pinus strobus*, pomegranate, *Ptychopetalum olacoides*, quinoa, red clover, rice, rosemary, rosemary oil, rooibos, rosehip, rosehip oil, safflower oil, *Saliconia herbacea*, *Scutellaria baicalensis*, shea butter, sunflower oil, *Symphytum officinale*, tamarind, tea, tea seed oil, *Theobroma grandiflorum*, tangerine, vanilla, vetiver oil, wheat	Arbutin, bisabolol, caffeine, coconut caprylic/capric triglyceride, ceramides, chrysin, citric acid, coco glycerides, hesperidin, linoleic acid, lysolecithin, phytosphingosine, plant glycerides, plant collagen, resveratrol, riboflavin, rice protein, salicylic acid, tocopherol, ubiquinone, ursolic acid, vegetable glycerin, vitamin C, whey protein

REFERENCES

1. Kanlayavattanakul M, Lourith N. An update on cutaneous aging treatment using herbs. J Cosmet Laser Ther. 2015;17:343–52.
2. Kanlayavattanakul M, Lourith N. Plants and natural products for the treatment of skin hyperpigmentation – a review. Planta Med. 2018;84:988–1006.
3. Sohm B, Cenizo V, André V, et al. Evaluation of the efficacy of a dill extract *in vitro* and *in vivo*. Int J Cosmet Sci. 2011;33:157–63.
4. Knott A, Reuschlein K, Mielke H, et al. Natural *Arctium lappa* fruit extract improves the clinical signs of aging skin. J Cosmet Dermatol. 2008;7:281–9.
5. Lee KK, Kim JH. Inhibitory effect of 150 plant extracts on elastase activity and their anti-inflammatory effects. Int J Cosmet Sci. 1999;21:71–82.
6. Lee KK, Choi JD. The effects of *Areca catechu* L. extract on anti-aging. Int J Cosmet Sci. 1999;21:285–95.
7. Chuarienthong P, Lourith N, Leelapornpisid P. Clinical efficacy comparison of anti-wrinkle cosmetics containing herbal flavonoids. Int J Cosmet Sci. 2010;32:99–106.
8. Frei B, Higdon JV. Antioxidant activity of tea polyphenols *in vivo*: evidence from animal studies. J Nutr. 2003;133:3275S–3284S.
9. Vayalil PK, Elmets CA, Katiyar SK. Treatment of green tea polyphenols in hydrophilic cream prevents UVB-induced oxidation of lipids and proteins, depletion of antioxidant enzymes and phosphorylation of MAPK proteins in SKH-1 hairless mouse skin. Carcinogenesis 2003;24:927–36.
10. Chung JH, Han JH, Hwang EJ, et al. Dual mechanisms of green tea extract (EGCG)-induced cell survival in human epidermal keratinocytes. FASEB J. 2003;17:1913–5.
11. Elmets CA, Singh D, Tubesing K, et al. Cutaneous photoprotection from ultraviolet injury by green tea polyphenols. J Am Acad Dermatol. 2001;44:425–32.
12. Haftek M, Mac-Mary S, Le Bitoux MA, et al. Clinical, biometric and structural evaluation of the long-term effects of a topical treatment with ascorbic acid and madecassoside in photoaged human skin. Exp Dermatol. 2008;17:946–52.
13. Lee J, Jung E, Kim Y, et al. Asiaticoside induces human collagen I synthesis through TGFβ receptor I kinase (TβRI kinase)-independent Smad signaling. Planta Med. 2006;72:324–8.
14. Lourith N, Kanlayavattanakul M. Formulation and clinical evaluation of the standardized *Litchi chinensis* extract for skin hyperpigmentation and aging treatments. Ann Pharm Fr. 2020;78:142–9.
15. Kim T, Lim HJ, Cho SK, et al. *Nelumbo nucifera* extracts as whitening and anti-wrinkle cosmetic agent. Korean J Chem Eng. 2011;28:424–427.
16. Mahmood T, Akhtar N. Combined topical application of lotus and green tea improves facial skin surface parameters. Rejuvenation Res. 2013;16:91–97.
17. Kanlayavattanakul M, Lourith N, Tadtong S, et al. Rice panicles: new promising unconventional cereal product for health benefits. J Cereal Sci. 2015;66:10–7.
18. Kanlayavattanakul M, Lourith N, Chaikul P. Jasmine rice panicle: a safe and efficient natural ingredient for skin aging treatments. J Ethnopharmacol. 2016;193:607–16.

19. Lee S, Lim JM, Jin MH, et al. Partially purified paeoniflorin exerts protective effects on UV-induced DNA damage and reduces facial wrinkles in human skin. J Cosmet Sci. 2006;57:57–64.
20. Kim YH, Chung CB, Kim JG, et al. Anti-wrinkle activity of zizyuglycoside I isolated from a *Sanguisorba officinalis* root extract and its application as a cosmeceutical ingredient. Biosci Biotechnol Biochem. 2008;72:303–11.
21. Matsumura Y, Ananthaswamy HN. Toxic effects of ultraviolet radiation on the skin. Toxicol Appl Pharmacol. 2004;195:298–308.
22. Rasul A, Akhtar N. Anti-aging potential of a cream containing milk thistle extract: formulation and *in vivo* evaluation. Afr J Biotechnol. 2012;11:1509–15.
23. Schmid D, Schürch C, Blum P, et al. Plant stem cell extract for longevity of skin and hair. SÖFW J. 2008;134:30–5.
24. Artaria C, Maramaldi G, Bonfigli A, et al. Lifting properties of the alkamide fraction from the fruit husks of *Zanthoxylum bungeanum*. Int J Cosmet Sci. 2011;33:328–33.
25. Khan BA, Akhtar N, Hussain I, et al. Whitening efficacy of plant extracts including *Hippophae rhamnoides* and *Cassia fistula* extracts on the skin of Asian patients with melisma. Postep Derm Alerfol. 2013;4:226–32.
26. Yamauchi K. Isolation, identification and tyrosinase inhibitory activities of the extractives from *Allamanda carthartica*. Nat Resour. 2011;2:167–72.
27. Yokota T, Nishio H, Kubota Y, et al. The inhibitory effect of glabridin from licorice extracts on melanogenesis and inflammation. Pigment Cell Res. 1998;11:355–61.
28. Amer M, Metwalli M. Topical liquiritin improves melisma. Int J Dermatol. 2000;39:299–301.
29. Koo J-H, Lee I, Yun S-K, et al. Saponified evening primrose oil reduces melanogenesis in B16 melanoma cells and reduced UV-induced skin pigmentation in humans. Lipids. 2010;45:401–7.
30. Kanlayavattanakul M, Chongnativisit W, Chaikul P, et al. Phenolic-rich pomegranate peel extract: *in vitro*, cellular, and *in vivo* activities for skin hyperpigmentation treatment. Planta Med. 2020; 86:749–59.
31. Kim MJ, Kim SM, Im KR, et al. Effect of hydroxycinnamic acid derivatives from corn bran on melanogenic protein expression. J Korean Soc Appl Biol Chem. 2010;53:422–6.
32. Kanlayavattanakul M, Lourith N. Biopolysaccharides for skin hydrating cosmetics. In: Ramawat KG, Mérillon J-M, eds, Polysaccharides. Switzerland: Springer; 2015: 1867–92.
33. Kanlayavattanakul M, Lourith N. Cosmetics: active polymers. In: Mirshra M, ed, Encyclopedia of polymer. Florida: CRC Press; 2019: 705–21.
34. Kanlayavattanakul M, Rodchuea C, Lourith N. Moisturizing effect of alcohol-based hand rub containing okra polysaccharide. Int J Cosmet Sci. 2012;34: 280–3.
35. Dal'Belo SE, Gaspar LR, Compos PMBGM. Moisturizing effect of cosmetic formulations containing *Aloe vera* extract in different concentrations assessed by skin bioengineering techniques. Skin Res Technol. 2006;12:241–6.
36. Lourith N, Kanlayavattanakul M. Ceylon spinach: a promising crop for skin hydrating products. Ind Crop Prod. 2017;105:24–8.

37. Kanlayavatanakul M, Pawakongbun P, Lourith N. Dendrobium orchid polysaccharide extract: preparation, characterization and *in vivo* skin hydrating efficacy. Chinese Herb Med. 2019;11:400–5.

38. Futrakul B, Kanlayavattanakul M, Krisdaphong P. Biophysic evaluation of polysaccharide gel from durian's fruit hulls for skin moisturizer. Int J Cosmet Sci. 2010;32:211–5.

39. Kanlayavattanakul M, Fungpaisalpong K, Pumcharoen M, et al. Preparation and efficacy assessment of malva nut polysaccharide for skin hydrating products. Ann Pharm Fr. 2017;75:436–45.

40. Pereda MDCV, Dieamant GDCD, Eberlin S, et al. Expression of differential genes involved in the maintenance of water balance in human skin by *Piptadenia colubrina* extract. J Cosmet Dermatol. 2010;9:35–43.

41. Eom SY, Chung CB, Kim YS, et al. Cosmeceutical properties of polysaccharides from the root bark of *Ulmus davidiana* var. *japonica*. J Cosmet Sci. 2006;57:355–67.

42. Kanlayavattanakul M, Lourith N. Therapeutic agents and herbs in topical application for acne treatment. Int J Cosmet Sci. 2011;33:289–97.

43. Meetham P. Kanlayavattanakul M, Lourith N. Development and clinical efficacy evaluation of anti-greasy green tea tonner on facial skin. Rev Bras Farmacogn. 2018;28: 214–7.

44. Raman A, Weir U, Bloomfield SF. Antimicrobial effects of tea tree oil and its major components on *Staphylococcus aureus*, *S. epidermidis* and *Propionibacterium acnes*. Lett App Microbiol. 1995;21:242–5.

45. Bassett IB, Pannowitz DL, Barnetson RS. A comparative study of tea tree oil versus benzoyl peroxide in the treatment of acne. Med J Aust. 1990;153:455–8.

46. Pongsakornpaisan P, Lourith N, Kanlayavattanakul M. Anti-sebum efficacy of guava toner: a split-face, randomized, single-blind placebo-controlled study. J Cosmet Dermatol. 2019;18:1737–41.

Phytocosmetics for Hair Care

5

Nattaya Lourith and
Mayuree Kanlayavattanakul

Contents

5.1 INTRODUCTION

Human hair plays an important role in social and sexual communication, with pronounced differences between ages and sexes, in addition to its protective function. Physical appearance and self-perception are crucially relied on, including, density and color of scalp hair. Graying of hair is dependent on the production of less pigment in the individual hairs with advancing age. Hair coloring products are therefore widely used both by men and women to alter natural hair color, postpone graying of hair, or restore pigmentation following graying [1]. Hair thinning and graying are important signs of aging accentuated by several factors.

Hair undergoes cyclic periods of growth – anagen, catagen, and telogen. The longest phase is anagen, varying between patients and body site. During hair growth phases, hair is differentiated into 2 types: vellus and terminal hairs. Vellus hair is thinner in diameter, shorter in length, lower in weight, and lighter in color than the terminal one. The anagen phase in scalp hair may last for longer than 3 years. At an early stage of anagen, vellus hair grows and changes into terminal hair, which is longer, thicker, and darker in color. Following the full development of terminal anagen, melanocyte diminishes in activity and melanin production eventually stops; keratinocyte no longer produces keratin fiber, shifting the hair into catagen, the intermediate phase. Consequently, the hair turns to telogen, the shedding phase, marked by hair lightening or grey hair and hair thinning (vellus hair), and finally loosening of hair from the scalp. In the meantime, the hair papilla prepares for new anagen hair generation [1, 2].

Male hormones, androgen, regulate vellus hair development into the terminal hair but function differently on the scalp. This male hormone regresses hair follicles, turning a terminal hair into vellus. That is widely recognized as male pattern baldness or androgenetic alopecia (AGA), the severity directly related to age. AGA is noticed as a slow transformation of large scalp terminal hair follicles into shorter, thinner, and less deep vellus hair with much shorter anagen. The mechanism is by a conversion of weak androgen – testosterone (T) – into 5α-dihydrotestosterone (DHT) by 5α-reductase, binding with androgen receptor (AR) and further transcription. Two isozymes of 5α-reductase, type I and type II, are well established for their actions in hair loss. In addition, dehydroepiandrosterone (DHEA) is metabolized into T, escalating hair loss [2, 3].

In addition to the direct effects of androgen on hair loss, greasiness of scalp, dryness of scalp, dandruff, and aging of hair (including grey hair) are indirect causes that make the degree of hair loss more severe. Excess sebum on the scalp produces the ideal environment for *Malassezia* spp., resulting in itching and dandruff and exacerbating hair loss via the accumulated oxidative stress in hair follicle and follicular micro-inflammation. Micro-inflammation escalates the severity of hair loss secondary to androgen. An anti-microbial agent not only suppresses the scalp normal flora accumulating in dandruff but can enhance hair rejuvenation with a reversal of the micro-inflammatory pathology [4]. Thus, an active with sebum reduction efficiency, limiting itching, would co-contribute to dandruff treatment in the same way inflammatory and microbial inhibitors are able to delay hair loss.

As addressed above, AGA is the outcome of combined factors and multifaceted actions of an active would suit the different etiologies of hair loss development. Nonetheless, anti-androgen actives are the ones mostly used and are the first ones examined in search of a promising treating agent. Although minoxidil and its derivatives (dutasteride and finasteride) are the most widely used agents for alopecia treatment, their undesired adverse effects encourage researching an alternative efficient treatment with limited side effects – particularly one from phytocosmetics.

5.2 PHYTOCOSMETICS FOR HAIR CARE

Phytocosmetic actives including minerals and vitamins (for instance, phytoestrogens and vitamin B) are associated with hair growth and strength. These agents efficiently delay grey hair or suppress hair loss by prolonging anagen and inducing activities and by shorting the telogen hair phase with a stimulating activity toward the proliferation of hair follicles and sustaining the cell age. The essential fatty acids – linolenic, linoleic, palmitoleic, oleic, myristoleic, and stearic acids – are known for their 5α-reductase inhibitory effect and hair regrowth promotion – particularly linolenic acid – with additional benefit for scalp hydration and maintaining homeostasis of the scalp condition with a low degree of greasiness and dandruff. In addition, phytosterols, phytoestrogens, phyto-derived fatty acids, and terpenoids prevent androgenetic mediated disorders by free radical scavenging and blocking the harmful effects of sex hormone reducing serum excretion/production. These phyto-actives are therefore capable of delaying the aging of hair, grey hair and hair loss, and are sufficiently accumulated on hair growth promotion to enhance hair loss prevention [2, 3].

This chapter therefore chiefly overviews those phytocosmetics that are potential treatments for hair loss, as well as those for greasy scalp, dandruff, and grey hair on the basis of scientific evidence, *in vitro*, cell culture models, and *in vivo,* as well as the phytocosmetic actives already recognized. Researchers may use this information for their further works to fill the gap in knowledge about phytocosmetics for hair care. Additionally, readers may optimize their choices of phytocosmetics to maintain healthy hair accordingly.

Saw palmetto (*Serenoa repens*), pygeum (*Pygeum africanum*), and stinging nettles (*Urtica dioica*) are commercialized as phytocosmetics combating hair loss. Saw palmetto, a 5α-reductase inhibitor [5], is commercialized in Permixon®, a lipido-sterolic extract containing high essential fatty acids content with phytosterols, β-carotene, and tocopherols, including β-sitosterol. This phytotherapeutic agent for hair loss treatment is very popular in Germany and France and has been shown to be effective without any enhancer [6–8]. Pygeum has been commercialized widely in Europe in Tadenan® [9] because it is a 5α-reductase inhibitor [10–11]. Stinging nettle was used as a traditional remedy in Europe and has been commercialized in many dosage forms [10] as it possess anti-androgenetic effects from its biologically active phenolics, fatty acids, phytosterols, and lignans [12, 13].

Asian traditional recipes are also documented for their uses against hair loss. Ayurvedic medicine formulation using *Cuscuta reflexa, Citrullus colocynthis*, and *Eclipta alba* potentially increase hair follicle number and scalp thickness, particularly by induction of anagen hair, comparing to minoxidil [14]. Creams comprising the herbs were evaluated on hair growth promoting efficacy in albino rats. The formulation exhibited a promising result in hair loss treatment [15]. Furthermore, there are other promising phytocosmetics for hair care, summarized next.

5.2.1 *Acacia concinna*

Natural saponin from *A. concinna* combines application in hair cleansing with additional benefit in anti-dandruff activity, inhibiting 21% of 5α-reductase at 200 μg/mL [16].

5.2.2 *Allium cepa*

Topical application of onion juice on the scalp was found to effective stimulate hair regrowth in both male and female [17]. This might be caused by its anti-inflammatory and anti-microbial effects due to its flavonoids [18, 19].

5.2.3 *Allium sativum*

Benign prostatic hyperplasia could be treated by garlic because of its anti-inflammatory and anti-oxidant effects [20]. In addition, it has been used to control dandruff owing to its anti-microbials [21].

5.2.4 *Aloe vera*

This gel had been traditionally used for hair loss and has been claimed to improve hair growth following alopecia [22] owing to aloenin, promoting hair growth without irritation [23], and also to its enrichment in multivitamin B [24].

5.2.5 *Artocarpus incisus*

The herb has shown potent 5α-reductase inhibitory activity [16], with constituents characterized as chlorophorin, artocarpin, and chalcone with IC_{50} of 37, 85, and 104 μm, respectively [25, 26].

5.2.6 *Asiasari radix*

This oriental medicine herb has been used for treating hair loss because it has hair growth promoting potential, stimulating transformation of telogen to anagen with induction of cellular proliferation [27].

5.2.7 *Camellia sinensis*

Tea has been continuously used and is well known as a daily beverage with pharmacological properties. Polyphenolic compounds in tea significantly increase hair regrowth [28]. Epigallocatechin-3-gallate, a main constituent of polyphenols in tea, has been reported to have potential against AGA by inhibition of 5α-reductase with hair growth enhancement [29, 30]. Tea was shown to be a safe and sufficient phytocosmetics for scalp greasiness treatment in 20 volunteers (10 female and 10 male, aged 23–35 years). Greasiness of the scalp was noted to be reduced from baseline at the first day of treatment and continued to reduce significantly below baseline after 21 and 28 days of application ($p = 0.024$ and 0.008) [31].

5.2.8 *Capsicum frutescens*

Capsaicin from chilies was found to accumulate in hair follicle, resulting in anagen induction, and promoted hair growth in volunteers with alopecia [32].

5.2.9 *Cimicifuga racemosa*

More potent inhibition of 5α-reductase than that caused by finasteride was reported for black cohosh extract [33].

5.2.10 *Cleistocalyx nervosum* var. *paniala* (*Syzygium nervosum* var. *paniala*)

This indigenous berry fruit with a sweet and sour taste contains health beneficial phenolics including the anthocyanins cyanidin-3-glucoside, cyanidin-5-glucoside, and cyanidin-3,5-diglucoside. The fruit anthocyanin standardized extract was prepared and formulated into hair coloring spray (7.46%) which met the panelists' preferences, stained hair efficiently, and persisted for more than five washes [34].

5.2.11 *Clitoria ternatea*

Butterfly pea has been used as a folk remedy against grey hair in Thailand. However, its activity against 5α-reductase is moderate, with only 29% of enzyme inhibited at an extract concentration of 200 µg/mL [16]. The stability of butterfly pea anthocyanins is enhanced when protected in the biopolymeric wall, with $12.04 \pm 4.49\%$ reduction of anthocyanins against $85.37 \pm 0.22\%$ reduction in the unprotected system. Furthermore, the particle size of the stabilized anthocyanins system was 95.44 ± 1.57 µm; this may be an important factor as the nano-carriers potentially boost potency of the anthocyanins [35].

5.2.12 *Citrus hystrix*

Kaffir lime is able to smoothe skin and suppress scalp dandruff with an exfoliation refreshing effect. It is a Thai folk remedy for hair loss, but has only moderate 5α-reductase inhibitory activity, albeit higher (25%) than *C. ternatea* at the same concentration [16].

5.2.13 *Cucurbita* spp.

Pumpkin contains several phytosterols that inhibit androgenetic mediated diseases [36]; its carotenoids and fatty acids suppress androgenetic expression as prostate cancer – particularly its high content of linoleic, oleic, palmitic, and stearic acids [37, 38].

5.2.14 *Cuscuta reflexa*

This traditional purgative herb in India exhibited hair growth promotion via a 5α-reductase inhibitory effect, albeit at lower potency than finasteride [39].

5.2.15 *Cymbopogon citratus* and *C. flexuosus*

The essential oil of West or East Indian lemongrass is widely used in pharmaceutical products. *C. flexuosus* oil inhibits *Malassezia furfur*, the major yeast associated with dandruff, at the minimum inhibitory concentration (MIC) of 6.70 ppm [40]. Lemongrass oil has been developed into anti-dandruff hair tonic (0%, 10%, and 15%) and its efficacy evaluated by a randomized, double-blind, placebo-controlled, split-head trial in 30 volunteers (20–60 years) experiencing dandruff. The volunteers applied the preparation twice daily for 14 consecutive days. Following the first week of treatment, lemongrass oil hair tonics significantly ($p < 0.05$) exhibited anti-dandruff efficacy and the efficacy was increased at the end of the study. In particular, 10% lemongrass oil hair tonic significantly ($p = 0.000$) reduced dandruff better than 5% and 15% formulas [41].

5.2.16 *Eclipta prostrata*

False daisy is a medicinal herb in Asian remedies for skin. This anti-inflammatory and anti-oxidant herb exhibited hair re-growth promotion in an animal model at a better activity than the control and minoxidil-treated groups. The anti-hair loss performance was confirmed in human dermal papilla cells; the activity of the extract at 10 µg/mL was comparable to 10 µm of minoxidil, while the extract at 50 µg/mL was significantly better than standard minoxidil [42].

5.2.17 *Ginkgo biloba*

This universal natural remedy has been used as a hair regrowth promoter with its epidermis growth stimulant, astringent, anti-inflammatory, and radical activities [43].

5.2.18 *Glycine max*

Soy protein – particularly soymetide-4 isolated from trypsin digestion – is another herbal product suppressing alopecia [44].

5.2.19 *Glycyrrhiza glabra*

Licorice was traditionally used for hair loss treatment, as it inhibits DHT formation, in addition to its anti-inflammatory effects from glycyrrhizin and glycyrrhetic acid [45].

5.2.20 *Junglan regia* and *J. nigra*

Walnuts were used to treat scalp itching and peeling relevant to dandruff, which accumulate in hair loss [46].

5.2.21 *Lawsonia inermis*

Henna – a herb coloring hair natural red shades – has been used as a hair growth accelerator since ancient times [47, 48].

5.2.22 *Panax ginseng*

A cell regeneration herb with anti-inflammatory and blood circulation effects, ginseng has also been used for skin and scalp treatment limiting hair loss [49]. The potential of ginseng extract to contribute to hair regeneration was again confirmed with cell proliferation improvement, including an *in vivo* efficacy evaluation in the mouse model with 1 mg/mL topical application on earlier anagen phase prolonging the mature anagen phase comparable to 5% minoxidil [50].

5.2.23 *Persea americana*

Avocado has been known for anti-itching and anti-dandruff properties that indirectly accumulate in hair loss; its ability to reduce sebum secretion could explain its anti-dandruff property. Furthermore, 5α-reductase type I was found to be deactivated by avocado. Biological activities of avocado, particularly against androgenetic expression [51], rely on its fatty acid constituents, vitamin B, and other biologically active compounds [52, 53].

5.2.24 *Phaseolus mungo*

Black bean is important as the second most consumed bean globally after soybean. It has been reported to be a sustainable source of anthocyanins, particularly delphinidin 3-glucoside, petunidin 3-glucoside, and malvidin 3-glucoside, known for pharmaceutic and cosmetic products. The standardized black bean anthocyanins were prepared and developed into hair coloring gel (10%), which was able to persist through at least four shampoo washes. Despite the natural anthocyanin property of dyeing hair only temporarily, this developed black bean hair coloring gel could be classified as a semi-permanent coloring gel based on its color staining ability. Adhesion of the coloring gel on the hair is enhanced by the contact time of the black bean anthocyanin extract, enabling penetration of the colorant molecules into the hair cuticle and partially diffusing throughout the cortex [54].

5.2.25 *Pulsatilla chinensis*

This herb is one of the important Chinese herbs for infectious disease treatment through its pharmacotherapeutically active saponins including betulinic acid, anemosapogenin, and hederagenin. The saponin extract (0.5 µg/mL) of the herb has demonstrated ability to diminish cellular inflammatory-induced stresses of human follicles and dermal papilla cells. In addition, the extract significantly increases pigmentation of the hair follicles isolated from the donors. The herb is therefore potentially to be used for stress-induced hair loss treatment [55].

5.2.26 *Rosmarinus officinalis*

Rosemary, reported to increase hair growth, was further evaluated for alopecia treatment. It stimulated hair growth with a reduction of sebum secretion, which made it additionally suitable for greasy hair treatment. Rosmarinic acids and other caffeic acid derivatives in rosemary are responsible for the biological activities through their anti-oxidant effects [56]. Furthermore, rosemary can be daily used for dandruff treatment.

5.2.27 *Roystonea regia*

Cuban royal palm has fatty acid enrichment that inhibits 5α-reductase [57–59].

5.2.28 *Salvia officinalis*

Sage in a combination with other herbs increased hair density. Sage itself was traditionally used for hair conditioning as it maintains the sheen of curly hair, and strengthens and stimulates hair growth, in addition to its abilities for dandruff, hair loss, and grey hair treatment [47].

5.2.29 *Sophora flavescens*

This herb is another oriental medicine for hair loss treatment, which has been proven to promote hair growth by it 5α-reductase type II inhibitory effect [60].

5.2.30 *Thuja occidentalis*

T. occidentalis was found to be a stronger 5α-reductase type II inhibitor than the standard linolenic acid [61].

5.2.31 *Vitis vinifera*

Grape seed contains many biologically active compounds including polyphenolic proanthocyanidins that consequently convert to procyanidins which possess a stronger anti-oxidative effect [62]. Proanthocyanidins from grape seeds stimulated hair follicle proliferation and accelerated hair converting from the telogen to the anagen phases [63].

5.2.32 *Zizyphus jujuba*

Its essential oil promoted hair length, diameter, and density following clinical evaluation in mice, particularly at 1% treatment. This hair promoting efficacy would be caused by fatty acid constituents, including palmitic, oleic, linoleic, linolenic, and arachidonic acids [64].

5.3 CONCLUSION

The benefits of phytocosmetics for hair loss treatment, the major market sector of hair care cosmetics, are summarized in Table 5.1. As multifunctional natural extracts/actives, some plants are revealed with additional hair benefits; many phytocosmetics for hair care are indicated for more than one indication out of dandruff, grey hair, and greasy hair treatments. In addition, some of these are incorporated in the commercialized products, e.g. those in the ingredient lists retrieved from the Amazon's best seller hair shampoos (Table 5.1). A mixture of ingredients can boost the performance of the preparation in terms

TABLE 5.1   Phytocosmetics for hair care

| NAME | | BENEFITS | | | |
SCIENTIFIC	COMMON	HAIR LOSS/ HAIR GROWTH	DANDRUFF	GREY HAIR	GREASY
Acacia concinna	Soap pod	✓			
Allium cepa	Onion	✓			
Allium sativum	Garlic		✓		
Aloe vera	Aloe	✓			
Artocarpus incisus	Breadfruit	✓			
Asiasari radix	Chinese wild ginger root	✓			
Camellia sinensis	Tea	✓			✓
Capsicum frutescens	Chili	✓			
Cimicifuga racemosa	Black cohosh	✓			
Citrullus colocynthis	Colocynth	✓			
Cleistocalyx nervosum	-			✓	
Clitoria ternatea	Butterfly pea	✓		✓	
Citrus hystrix	Kaffir lime	✓			
Curcubita spp.	Pumpkin	✓			
Cuscuta reflexa	giant dodder	✓			
Cymbopogon citratus	Lemongrass		✓		
Eclipta spp.	False daisy	✓			
Ginkgo biloba	Ginkgo	✓			
Glycine max	Soy	✓			
Glycyrrhiza glabra	Licorice	✓			
Junglan spp.	Walnut	✓	✓		
Lawsonia inermis	Henna	✓		✓	
Panax ginseng	Ginseng	✓			
Persea americana	Avocado	✓	✓		✓

TABLE 5.1 (*Continued*)

	NAME	BENEFITS			
		HAIR LOSS/		GREY	
SCIENTIFIC	COMMON	HAIR GROWTH	DANDRUFF	HAIR	GREASY
Phaseolus mungo	Black bean			✓	
Pulsatilla chinensis	Bai Tou Weng			✓	
Pygeum africanum	Pygeum	✓			
Rosmarinus officinalis	Rosmary	✓			
Roystonea regia	Cuban royal palm	✓			
Salvia officinalis	Sage	✓	✓	✓	
Serenoa repens	Saw palmeto	✓			
Thuja occidentalis	Eastern white cedar	✓			
Urtica dioica	Stinging nettle	✓			
Vitis vinifera	Grape	✓			
Zizyphus jujuba	Jujube	✓			

Phytocosmetic ingredients

EXTRACT	ACTIVE
Aloe, amla oil, argan oil, black cumin seed, black cumin seed oil, coconut oil, evening primrose oil, green tea, hemp oil, jojoba oil, mango butter, nettle, olive oil, peppermint oil, *Polygonum multiflorum*, pygeum, rosmary oil, saw palmetto, tea tree oil	Phytokeratin, caffeine, menthol

of safety, efficacy, stability, and consumer preferences. The key success factors for phyto-actives are preparation of the actives and specification of the quality profiles (i.e. chemical and biological profiles including toxicology, stability, and compatibility with the available cosmetic raw materials and packaging). In addition, consumer enthusiasm for phytocosmetic products is to be noted. It will be a key challenging area for researchers for create and develop phytocosmetics for hair care in line with the information presented here.

REFERENCES

1. Robbins CR. Chemical and physical behavior of human hair. New York: Springer; 2002.
2. Lourith N, Kanlayavattanakul M. Hair loss and herbs for treatment. J Cosmet Dermatol. 2013;12:210–2.
3. Lourith N, Kanlayavattanakul M. Herbal treatment for hair loss and alopecia: an overview. In: Bagchi D, Preuss HG, Swaroop A, eds, Nutraceuticals and functional foods in human health and disease prevention. Florida: CRC Press; 2015: 475–82.
4. Pierard GF, Pierard-Franchimont C, Nikkels-Tassiudji N, et al. Improvement in the inflammatory aspect of androgenetic alopecia. A pilot study with an antimicrobial lotion. J Dermatol Treat. 1996;7:153–7.
5. Palin MF, Faguy M, LeHoux JG, et al. Inhibitory effects of *Serenoa repens* on the kinetic of pig prostatic microsomal 5α-reductase activity. Endocrine. 1998;9:65–9.
6. Schantz MM, Bedner M, Long SE, et al. Development of saw palmetto (*Serenoa repens*) fruit and extract standard reference materials. Anal Bioanal Chem. 2008;392:427–38.
7. Bedner M, Schantz MM, Sander LC, et al. Development of liquid chromatographic methods for the determination of phytosterols in standard reference materials containing saw palmetto. J Chromatogr A. 2008;1192:74–80.
8. Debruyne F, Koch G, Boyle P, et al. Comparison of a phytotherapeutic agent (Perximon) with an α-blocker (tamsulosin) in the treatment of benign prostatic hyperplasia: a 1 year randomised international study. Eur Urol. 2002;41:497–507.
9. Ishani A, MacDonald R, Nelson D, et al. *Pygeum africanum* for the treatment of patient with benign prostatic hyperplasia: a systematic review and quantitative meta-analysis. Am J Med. 2000;109:654–64.
10. Hartman RW, Mark M, Soldati F. Inhibition of 5α-reductase and aromatase by PHL-00801 (Prostatonin), a combination of PY 102 (*Pygeum africanum*) and UR 102 (*Urtica dioica*) extracts. Phytomedicine. 1996;4:121–8.
11. Rodes L, Primka RL, Berman C, et al. Comparison of finasteride (Proscar), a 5α-reductase inhibitor and various commercial plant extracts *in vitro* and *in vivo* 5α-reductase inhibition. Prostate 1993;22:43–51.
12. Levin RM, Das AK. A scientific basis for the therapeutic effects of *Pygeum africanum* and *Serenoa repens*. Urol Res. 2000;28:201–9.
13. Chrubasik JE, Roufogalis BD, Wagner H, et al. A comprehensive review on the stinging nettle effect and efficacy profiles. Part II: *Urticae radix*. Phytomedicine. 2007;14:568–79.
14. Datta K, Singh AT, Mukherjee A, et al. *Eclipta alba* extract with potential for hair growth promoting activity. J Ethanopharmacol. 2009;124:450–6.
15. Roy RK, Thakur M, Dizxt VK. Development and evaluation of polyherbal formulation for hair growth-promoting activity. J Cosmet Dermatol. 2007;6:108–12.
16. Shimizu K, Kondo R, Sakai K, et al. U. 5α-Reductase inhibitory component from leaves of *Artocarpus altilis*. J Wood Sci. 2000;46:385–9.

17. Sharquie KE. Onion juice (*Allium cepa* L.), a new topical treatment for alopecia areata. J Dermatol. 2002;29:343–6.
18. Dorsch W. *Allium cepa* L. (onion). Part 2: chemistry, analysis and pharmacology. Phytomedicine. 1996;3:391–7.
19. Griffiths G, Trueman L, Crowther T, Thomas B, Smith B. Onions – a global benefit to health. Phytother Res. 2002;16:603–15.
20. Devrim E, Durak I. Is gallic a promising food for benign prostatic hyperplasia and prostate cancer? Molec Nutr Food Res. 2007;51:1319–23.
21. Ariga T, Seki T. Flavor components of garlic (*Allium sativum* L.) and their multiple functions. Aroma Res. 2000;1:16–27.
22. Grindlay D, Reynolds T. The *Aloe vera* phenomenon: a review of the properties and modern uses of the leaf parenchyma gel. J Ethanopharmacol. 1986;16:117–51.
23. Inaoka Y, Fukushima M, Kuroda H. Hair tonics containing aloenin. Jpn Kokai Tokkyo Koho. 1988; 3: JP63198615.
24. Davis RH, DiDonato JJ, Hartman GM, Hass RC. Antiinflammatory and wound healing activity of a growth substance in *Aloe vera*. J Am Podiatr Med Assoc. 1994;84:77–81.
25. Shimizu K, Fukuda M, Kondo R, Sakai K. The 5α-reductase inhibitory components from heartwood of *Artocarpus incisus*: structure-activity investigations. Planta Med. 2000;66:16–9.
26. Shimizu K, Kondo R, Sakai K, Buabarn S, Dilokkunanant U. A geranylated chalcone with 5α-reductase inhibitory properties from *Artocapus incisus*. Phytochemistry. 2000;54:737–9.
27. Rho SS, Park SJ, Hwang SL, et al. The hair growth promoting effect of *Asiasari radix* extract and its molecular regulation. J Dermatol Sci. 2005;38:89–97.
28. Esfandiari A, Kelley P. The effects of tea polyphenolic compounds on hair loss among rodents. J Natl Med Assoc. 2005;97:816–8.
29. Hiipakka RA, Zhang HZ, Dai W, et al. Structure-activity relationships for inhibition of human 5α-reductase by polyphenol. Biochem Pharmacol. 2002;63:1165–76.
30. Kwon OS, Han JH, Yoo HG, et al. Human hair growth enhancement *in vitro* by green tea epigallocatechin-3-gallate (EGCG). Phytomedicine. 2007;14:551–5.
31. Nualsri C, Lourith N, Kanlayavattanakul M. Development and clinical evaluation of green tea hair tonic for greasy scalp treatment. J Cosmet Sci. 2016;67:161–6.
32. Harada N, Okajima K, Arai M, et al. Administration of capsaicin and isoflavone promotes hair growth by increasing insulin-like growth factor-I production in mice and humans with alopecia. Growth Horm IGF Res. 2007;17:408–15.
33. Sedlová-Wuttke D, Pitzel L, Thelen P, Wuttke W. Inhibition of 5α-reductase in the rat prostate by *Cimicifuga racemosa*. Maturitas. 2006;55:S75–82.
34. Pipattanamomgkol P, Lourith N, Kanlayavattanakul M. The natural approach to hair dyeing product with *Cleistocalyx nervosum* var. *paniala*. Sustain Chem Pharm. 2018;8:88–93.
35. Lourith N, Kanlayavattanakul M. Improved stability of butterfly pea anthocyanins with biopolymeric walls. J Cosmet Sci. 2020;71:1–10.
36. Carbin BE, Larsson B, Lindahl O. Treatment of benign prostatic hyperplasia with phytosterols. Br J Urol. 1990;66,636–41.
37. Hodge AM, English DR, McCredie MRE, et al. Food, nutrients and prostate cancer. Cancer Causes Control. 2004;15:11–20.

38. Nesterova OV, Samylina IA, Bobylev RV, et al. Study of physicochemical properties and fatty acid composition of pumkin oil. Farmatsiya. 1990;39:75–6.
39. Pandit S, Chauhan NS, Dixit VK. Effect of *Cuscuta reflexa* Roxb on androgen-induced alopecia. J Cosmet Dermatol. 2008;7:199–204.
40. Galuppo R, Aureli S, Bonoli C, et al. Effectiveness of essential oils against Malassezia spp.: comparison of two *in vitro* tests. Mikologia Lekarska. 2010;17:79–84.
41. Chaisripipat W, Lourith N, Kanlayavattanakul M. Anti-dandruff hair tonic containing lemongrass (*Cymbopogon flexuosus*) oil. Forsch Komplementmed. 2015;22:226–9.
42. Lee K-H, Choi D, Jeong S-I, et al. *Elipta prostrata* promotes the induction of anagen, sustains the anagen phase trough regulation of FGF-7 and FGF-5. Pharm Biol. 2019;57:105–11.
43. Kobayashi N, Suzuki R, Koide C, et al. Effect of leaves of *Ginkgo biloba* on hair regrowth in C3H strain mice. Yagugaku Zasshi. 1993;113:718–24.
44. Tsuruki T, Takahata K, Yoshikawa M. Anti-alopecia mechanisms of soymetide-4, an immunostimulating peptide derived from soy β-conglycini. Peptides. 2005;26:707–11.
45. Olukoga A, Donaldson D. Historical perspectives on health. The history of liquorice: the plant, its extract, cultivation, commercialization and etymology. J R Soc Health. 1998;118:300–4.
46. Bruneton J, Pharmacognosy, phytochemistry, medicinal plants. Paris: Lavoisier Publishing; 1999.
47. Dweck AC. African plants. Cosmet Toilet. 1997;112:41–51.
48. Ali BH, Bashir AK, Tanira MOM. Anti-inflammatory, anti-pyretic and analgesic effects of *Lawsonia inermis* L. (henna) in rats. Pharmacology. 1995;51:356–63.
49. Kim SH, Jeong KS, Ryu SY, et al. *Panax ginseng* prevents apoptosis in hair follicles and accelerates recovery of hair medullary cells in irradiated mice. In Vivo. 1998;12:219–2.
50. Park S, Shin W-S, Ho J. *Fructus panax ginseng* extract promotes hair regeneration in C57BL/6 mice. J Ethnoparmacol. 2011;138:340–4.
51. Lu QY, Arteaga JR, Zhang Q, et al. Inhibition of prostate cancer cell growth by avocado extract: role of lipid-soluble bioactive substances. J Nutr Biochem. 2005;16:23–30.
52. Vilson JA, Su X, Zubik L, Bose P. Phenols antioxidant quantity and quality in foods: fruit. J Agric Food Chem. 2001;49:5315–21.
53. Domergue F, Helms GL, Prusky D, Browse J. Antifungal compounds from idioblast cells isolated from avocado fruit. Phytochemistry. 2000;54:183–9.
54. Inman C, Lourith N, Kanlayavattanakul M. Alternative application approach on black bean: hair coloring product. Chem Biol Technol Agric. 2020;7. doi:10.1186/s40538-019-0163-2.
55. Nam YJ, Lee EY, Choi E-J, et al. CRH receptor antagonists from *Pulsatilla chinensis* prevent CRH-induced premature catagen transition in human hair follicles. J Cosmet Dermatol. 2020;00:1–9. doi:10.1111/jocd.13328.
56. Aruoma OI, Spencer JP, Rossi R, et al. An evaluation of the antioxidant and antiviral action of extracts of rosemary and provençal herbs. Food Chem Toxicol. 1996;34:449–56.

57. Arruzazabala ML, Carbajal D, Mas R, et al. Preventive effects of D-004, a lipid extract from Cuban royal palm (*Rostonea regia*) fruits on testosterone-induced prostate hyperplasia in intact and castrated rodents. Drugs Exp Clin Res. 2004;30:227–33.

58. Cabajal D, Arruzazabala ML, Mas R, et al. Effects of D-004, a lipid extract from Cuban royal palm fruit on inhibiting prostatic hypertrophy induced with testosterone or dihydrotestosterone in a rat model: a randomized, controlled study. Curr Ther Res Clin Exp. 2004;65:505–14.

59. Perez LY, Menendez R, Mas R, Gonzalez RM. *In vitro* effect of D-004, a lipid extract of the fruit of the Cuban royal palm (*Roystonea regia*) on prostate steroid 5α-reductase activity. Curr Ther Res. 2006;67:396–405.

60. Roh SS, Kim CD, Lee MH, et al. The hair growth promoting effect of *Sophora flavescens* extract and its molecular regulation. J Dermatol Sci. 2002;30:43–9.

61. Park WS, Lee CH, Lee BG, et al. The extract of *Thujae occidentalis* semen inhibited 5alpha-reductase and androchronogenetic alopecia of B6CBAF1/j hybrid mouse. J Dermatol Sci. 2003;31:91–8.

62. Pietta P, Simometti P, Mauri P. Antioxidant activity of selected medicinal plants. J Agric Food Chem. 1998;46:4487–90.

63. Takahashi T, Kamiya T, Yoko Y. Proanthocyanidins from grape seeds promote proliferation of mouse hair follicle cells *in vitro* and convert hair cycle *in vivo*. Acta Derm Venereol. 1998;78:428–32.

64. Yoon JI, Al-Reza SM, Kang SC. Hair growth promoting effect of *Zizyphus jujuba* essential oil. Food Chem Tox. 2010;48:1350–4.

Phytocosmetics for Malodor Treatment

6

Nattaya Lourith and Mayuree Kanlayavattanakul

Contents

6.1 INTRODUCTION

Body odors – i.e. axillary and foot odor – can embarrass and impair self-confidence. Deodorant, anti-perspirant, and fragrance products are therefore popularly applied for unpleasant body odor suppression and masking. Bad breath or oral malodor is also a significant problem. Accordingly, the global consumption of mouth rinses is increasing, as well as other kinds of oral odor care products claiming to mask or prevent bad breath. Malodorant treatment products are therefore reckoned to be a multibillion dollar section of the cosmetic and personal care industries. In addition, those of odorless cosmetics are highly in demand among those consumers who are sensitive to odor; odor masking agents are therefore widely used for this application and among these, those of phyto-derived products are of popular interest. This chapter chiefly concerns malodor treatment with phytocosmetic actives; body and oral malodorants are addressed with their causes only briefly, as their causes are exhaustively detailed elsewhere [1, 2].

6.1.1 Body Malodorants

Human scent is genetically controlled and systemically influenced by dietary and medicinal intake, as well as by fragrance product application. Heavy sweating or hyperhidrosis, particularly at axillary sites, leads to unpleasant odors; adolescence can exacerbate sweat and consequent malodorant production [1].

Hyperhidrosis causes extreme body malodor known as osmidrosis, bromhidrosis, or offensive body odor. During the course of hyperhidrosis, an excellent environment for the growth of cutaneous microorganisms is provided, especially the malodorant generating species i.e. aerobic cocci of the *Micrococcaceae* family, aerobic diphtheroids (mainly *Corynebacterium*), anaerobic diphtheroids (*Propionibacterium*), and yeast (*Pityrosporum*). Thereafter, malodorous acids, steroids, and thiols are abundantly produced. The characteristic body malodorous acids are (*E*)-3-methyl-2-hexenoic acid (3M2H) and 3-hydroxy-3-methyl hexanoic acid (HMHA). Foot odor is mostly due to short-chain fatty acids i.e. acetic, propionic, butyric, isobutyric, valeric, isovaleric, and isocaproic acids. Malodorous steroids are androstenone (5α-androst-16-en-3-one) and androstenol (5α-androst-16-en-3α-ol). Body malodorous thiols are 3-sulphanylhexanol (3SH), 2-methyl-3-sulphanylbutanol (2M3SB), 3-sulphanylpentanol (3SP), and 3-sulphanylalkanol (particularly 3-methyl-3-sulphanyl hexanol; 3M3SH). Biosynthesis, translocations, and ventilation of these body malodorants are summarized in the literature [1].

6.1.2 Oral Malodorants

Oral malodor or halitosis is caused by several factors, including microorganisms causing odorous degradation substances derived from food and medicinal intakes, oral hygiene behavior, and respiratory conditions. The characteristic oral malodorants are volatile sulfur and nitrogen compounds (VSCs and VNCs), the degradation products of amino acids containing sulfur such as cysteine, cystine, and methionine. Amino acids are catabolized by oral anaerobes i.e. *Treponema denticola, Porphyromonas gingivalis, Prevotella intermedia, Bacteroides forsythus, Fusobacterium nucleatum, Porphyromonas endodontalis* and *Tannerella forsythensis* and tongue coating bacteria such as *Veillonella, Actinomyces,* and *Prevotella* species. The catabolism processes produce hydrogen sulfide (H_2S), methyl mercaptan (CH_3SH), cadaverine, putrescine, indole, and amines. In addition, fatty acids such as acetic acid, propionic acid, butyric acid, and isovaleric acid also contribute to exhaled bad breath. Other compounds produced during physical illness which accumulate in bad breath are ketonic compounds, acetone, methylethylketone, *n*-propanol, the heterocyclic compounds aniline and *o*-toluidine, and the nitrogen compounds dimethylamine and trimethylamine (CH_3N). Thus, several volatile organic compounds (VOCs) accumulate in bad breath; H_2S and CH_3SH are mainly diagnostic for oral malodor [2].

In regards with the production of malodorants, the active ingredients especially Zn salts are common in commercialized products, as well as Mn salts and those of anti-microbial agents i.e. Ag salts, triclosan, and cetyl pyridinium chloride, etc. [1, 2]. Nonetheless, potentially safe and efficient phyto-actives combating malodor are increasing. Those phytocosmetics capable and available to be used as safe and efficient malodorant treatments are summarized next.

6.2 PHYTOCOSMETICS FOR BODY MALODOR TREATMENT

Phytocosmetic actives are applicable for body odor treatment through their inhibitory effect against malodorant producing microbes. Flavonoids are one of the important actives with deodorizing effects. Thanks to their structural 3',4'-hydroxyl units with the additional 5,7-dihydroxyl groups that boost antimicrobial activity [3], they additionally possess an inhibitory effect in different malodorant producing pathways against androgen receptor.

Several traditional remedies are documented for body odor control. Kampo formulation containing *Rehmanniae radix*, *Cnidii rhizoma*, *Angelicae radix*, *Scutellariae radix* (17%, each) and *Phellodendri cortex*, *Coptidis rhizoma*, and *Gardenae fructus* (8%, each) was found to suppress *P. avidum* activity, significantly reducing the production of butyric acid (p = 0.047) [4]. Furthermore, the common spices rosemary (*Rosmarinus officinalis*) and sage (*Salvia officinalis*) were comparatively examined on their potency against malodorants generated by *S. epidermidis* and *Corynebacterium* spp. Rosemary was shown to be a better anti-microbial herb than sage with MIC (minimum inhibitory concentration) of 10 and 2 ppm, and 20 and 10–20 ppm, respectively [5]. Essential oils of oregano (*Origanum minutiflorum* and *O. onites*), black thyme (*Thymbra spicata*), and savory (*Satureja cuneifolia*), containing cavracrol, were shown to inhibit *C. xerosis* at the dilution range of 1:50–1:200 [6]. Cumin (*Cuminum cyminum*), sweet fennel (*Foeniculum vulgare*), laurel (*Laurus nobilis*), mint (*Mentha spicata*), marjoram (*O. majorana*), pickling herb (*Echinophoria tenuifoli*), sage (*Salvia aucheri*), and thyme (*T. sintenesi*) oils were found to inhibit *C. xerosis* at the oil concentration of 0.2–2% [7]. Cavacrol was proved to be the major active constituent that inhibited *S. epidermidis* at an MIC of 0.22 µl (of 70% carvacrol solution in methanol) [8]. In addition to these promising herbs, other phytocosmetic sources are summarized next.

6.2.1 *Abies cilicica*

Essential oil of Cilician fir potently inhibited *C. xerosis* with an MIC of 1.5 ppm. Limonene was the most potent inhibitor with MIC of 3 ppm, while α- and β-pinene as well as myrcene had an MIC of greater than 8 ppm [9].

6.2.2 *Allium sativum*

Garlic possesses anti-bacterial activity, including *S. epidermidis* inhibition. *S. epidermidis* (90–93%) was killed by garlic in 1 h, although resistance was found following 3–4 h of incubation [10]. In spite of the availability and low cost of garlic extraction and production, its pungent active sulfur compounds are an obstacle to its application. Preparation of the selected active principle with a suppressed odor of the extract might exclude those active sulfur molecules. The optimized delivery system with a controlled releasing rate, balancing with the phyto-active odor with its activity, would be a better solution for use of garlic in cosmetic and personal care products.

6.2.3 *Arctopus* spp.

This flowering plant is endemic to South African where it is counted as one of the most important medicinal herbs. Its phytocosmetic appreciation comes from its anti-microbial activity against *S. epidermidis*, which is better than standard ciprofloxacin (MIC = 600 ppm). *A. monacanthus* was exhibited as the strongest variety, followed by *A. echinatus* and *A. dregei* (MIC = 20–50, 50–200, and 100–900 ppm), respectively [11].

6.2.4 *Boswellia serrata*

The Indian frankincense tree posed a stronger activity against *Corynebacterium* spp. (MIC = 1–10 ppm), but was moderate against *S. epidermidis* (MIC = 100 ppm). (+)-Usnic and carnosic acids were revealed as the anti-microbial agents with a stronger activity than the extract. (+)-usnic acid inhibited *S. epidermidis* at an MIC of 4 ppm and *Corynebacterium* spp. at 4–8 ppm, whereas those of carnosic acid were 64 and 32–64 ppm, respectively [5].

6.2.5 *Camellia sinensis*

Tea can be reckoned as the universal herb with several cosmetic benefits, including for malodorant treatment. Tea gallocatechins and their gallates have been claimed as the main constituents responsible for anti-bacterial activity [12] with MBC (minimum bactericidal concentration) and MIC of 550 and 410 ppm. In addition, tea's effect on androgen receptors [13] synergistically prevented and reduced body malodor.

6.2.6 *Chaenomeles speciosa*

This herb had been documented in several East Asian traditional recipes (e.g. Chinese medicine, zhou pi mugua). This evergreen-shrub with red or white or pink flower is commonly called flowering quince, Chinese quince, or Japanese quince. It has been used in a form of essential oil for anti-microbial, anti-inflammatory, and anti-tumor properties with hepatoprotective effects. The pharmacological activities of the herb are determined by its β-caryophyllene (12.52%) and linalool (1.33%) constituents. In addition, it moderately inhibited *S. epidermidis* (MIC and MBC of 1,570 and 3,130 ppm) in a comparison with levofloxacin (MIC = 610, MBC = 1,220 ppm) [14].

6.2.7 *Coriandrum sativum*

Coriander oil inhibits micrococci and diphtheroids at an MIC of 0.1% due to its oxygenated terpenoids. Coriander oil could be incorporated into a stick deodorant at 1.0–6.0% w/w, although the preferred amount was 1.8–2.2% w/w. This formulation absorbed moisture [15], thereby inhibiting microbial metabolism.

6.2.8 *Gunnera perpensa*

This African traditional medicinal herb has been used for psoriasis. Its isolated pure compounds were shown to have inhibitory effect against malodorant generating microbe *S. epidermidis*. However, the isolated benzopyran (2-methyl-6-(3-methyl-2-butenyl)benzo-1,4-quinone and 6-hydroxy-8-methyl-2,2-dimethyl-2H-benzopyran) inhibited *S. epidermidis* at a weaker activity than standard ciprofloxacin (MIC = 9.8, 187, and 1.25 ppm, respectively) [16].

6.2.9 *Glycyrrhiza glabra*

Licorice root extract has been used to formulate aerosol, roll-on, powder, cream, lotion, stick, and detergent deodorants to control axillary odor. The active ingredient, glycyrrhetinic acid, is effective at a concentration of 0.01 to 5% w/w. The preparation comprises tannic acid, resorcin, phenol, sorbic acid, and salicylic acid, with odor-masking agents (musk, skatole, lemon oil, lavender oil, absolute jasmine, vanillin, benzoin, benzyl acetate, and menthol) [17].

6.2.10 *Harpagophytum procumbens*

Devil's claw had been shown as one of the potential herbs to use against malodorant generating microbes (MIC = 10 ppm; *S. epidermidis* and 10–20 ppm; *Corynebacterium* spp.) [5].

6.2.11 *Harungana madagascariensis*

Dragon's blood tree is well known for its topical anti-bacterial properties and has been used to treat cutaneous mycoses because of its biologically active flavonoids, alkaloids, saponins, glycosides, and tannins [18]. The herb was found to inhibit armpit and foot odor-producing bacteria with MIC and MBC ranges of 25–250 and 100–750 ppm, respectively. Furthermore, *C. xerosis* was killed at 200 ppm, whereas the growth of *S. epidermidis* was inhibited at 250 ppm. This effect was clearly mediated by flavanones (i.e. astilbin or 3-O-α-L-rhamnoside-5,7,3',4'-tetrahydroxydihydroflavonol) [19].

6.2.12 *Hibicus sabdariffa*

Hawaiian rose with *S. epidermidis* inhibitory activity (MIC = 625 ppm) [15] has been formulated into deodorant products [20].

6.2.13 *Humulus lupulus*

Hop is one of the promising anti-microbial herbs for use against odorant-producing bacteria. The herbal activity against *C. xerosis* was more noticeable (MIC and MBC of 6.25 and 25 ppm) than against *S. epidermidis* (MIC and MBC of 25 and > 25 ppm). Deodorant-containing hop extract (0.2%) was formulated accordingly and was found to inhibit *C. xerosis* four times stronger than *S. epidermidis* (inhibition zone of 8 and 2 mm, respectively). In addition, axillary malodor decreased from 6.28 ± 0.70 to 1.80 ± 0.71, 1.82 ± 0.74, and 2.24 ± 0.77 following 8, 12, and 24 h of application, respectively [21].

6.2.14 *Melaleuca alternifolia*

Tea tree oil has also been used in deodorants because of terpinen-4-ol, the active anti-microbial agent. MIC and MBC of the oil against *Corynebacterium* spp. were 0.5 and 2% (v/v), respectively. In addition, it inhibits *Staphylococcus* spp. at an MIC and MBC of 0.5 and 1–2% (v/v), respectively – in particular, *S. epidermidis* (MIC = 0.5% and MBC = 2% v/v) [22].

6.2.15 *Prunus armeniaca*

Apricot (500 ppm) was shown to inhibit >95% of androstenone generation following an incubation of androsterone sulfate with *C. xerosis*. The suppressive effect of androstenone was also exhibited at lower concentrations (125 and 62.5 ppm). Apricot was more effective than triclosan, which was used as a positive control [23].

6.2.16 *Sideritis* spp.

Essential oils from two cultivars of ironwort or mountain tea, traditionally used as herbal medicine, were evaluated on *S. epidermidis*. *S. cedretorum* showed stronger *S. epidermidis* inhibition than *S. erythrantha*, and better than standard vancomycin (10.00 ± 0.24 mm at 10 µl and 10.00 ± 0.24 mm at 30 µg). The activity was ruled by the volatile compounds, pulegone and linalool [24].

6.2.17 *Smyrniopsis aucheri*

Essential oil of *S. aucheri* containing α-bisabolol (19.91%), α- and β-pinene (15.10% and 6.58%), is widely used in cosmetics, including underarm deodorants. The oil was found to potently inhibit *S. epidermidis* [25].

6.2.18 *Satureja* spp.

Essential oils of *S. masukensis* potently inhibit *S. epidermidis*, followed by *S. pseudosimensis* and *S. biflora* (MIC = 370, 750, and 980 ppm, respectively).

Linalool has been shown to be the major aroma constituent of *S. masukensis* oil (4.44%) and was found to be the strongest inhibitor against *S. epidermidis* (MIC = 250 ppm), compared to caryophyllene oxide and pulegone (MIC = 900 and 950 ppm, respectively); the anti-biotics amoxicillin with clavulanic acid and netilmicin had an MIC of 3 and 4 ppm, respectively [26].

6.2.19 *Tamarix ramosissima*

Salt cedar has long been used as traditional astringent and tonic herb. The herb, rich in tannins and phenolics, potently inhibited *C. diphtheria* at an MIC of 25 ppm [27].

6.2.20 *Terminalia* spp.

T. ferdinandiana has been shown as the most potent cultivar against *C. jeikeium*, followed by *T. chebula*, *T. carpentariae*, and *T. sericea* (MIC = 233, 384, 450, and 549 ppm). *S. epidermidis* was greatly inhibited by *T. chebula*, *T. ferdinandiana*, *T. carpentariae*, and *T. sericea* (MIC = 187, 220, 295, and 383 ppm). The growth of *P. acnes* was highly suppressed by *T. chebula*, *T. carpentariae*, *T. sericea*, and *T. ferdinandiana* (MIC = 478, 500, 514, and 625 ppm). These tropical plants are therefore highlighted as promising sources against body malodorant producing microbes due to their tannins and flavones contents, especially those of Terminalia phyto-actives chebulic, chebulagic, and chebulinic acids, including ellagic acid and corilagin as examined by LC/MS [28, 29].

6.2.21 *Ziziphora* spp.

Z. clinopodioides oil contains (+)-pulegone (31.86%) 1,8-cineole (12.21%), and limonene (10.48%) as the major aroma compounds and inhibit *Corynebacterium* spp. at an MIC of 15.60–31.25 ppm [30]. *S. epidermidis* is moderately inhibited by the essential oil with an MIC of 60–1,000 ppm [31]. In addition, *Z. persica* oil containing high levels of (+)-pulegone (79.33%) but low levels of limonene (6.78%) exhibit a wide range of *Corynebacterium* spp. inhibition (MIC = 250–7.81 ppm).

Generally, a mixture of herbs or phytocosmetics is commonly used against bad odor. A mixture of *Camellia sinensis*, *Hibicus sabdariffa*, *Malva sylvestris*, *Vitis viticola*, *Daucus carota*, *Commiphora myrrh*, *Simmondsia chinensis*, and *Calendula officinalis* has been incorporated into deodorant aerosols, gels, emulsions, sticks, creams, powders, soaps, and lotions [20].

Ginkgo biloba leaf and *Phellodendron amurense* bark extracts were effectively used as deodorants at 0.1–20% w/w, although the most commonly used amount was 0.5–10% w/w [32].

6.3 PHYTOCOSMETICS FOR ORAL MALODOR TREATMENT

The volatility of methyl mercaptan can be reduced by betel leaves (*Piper betel*), which are used to treat halitosis [33, 34]. The anti-microbial phenolic compound in betel leaves was identified as allylpyrocatechol [34]. Other phenolic compounds inhibiting oral microbes and reducing bad breath are catechin and resveratrol extracted from licorice (*Glycyrrhiza* spp.), *Camellia* spp., *Acacia catechu*, *Polygonum* spp., *Areca catechu*, *Potentilla fragarioides*, Rheum, Prunus, *Ginkgo biloba*, Machilus, Elaeagnus, Apocynum, and Geranium [35] including phytic acid [36]. In addition, a herbal formulation of *Echinacea angustifolia*, *Pistacia lentiscus*, lavender (*Lavendula angustifolia*), and sage (*Salvia officinalis*) extracts was found to be effective against oral malodor [37]. In addition to anti-microbial efficacies in these plant extracts, their aromatic effects are appreciable for bad breath neutralization and flavoring the treatment products.

With bactericidal activity against dental pathogenic microorganisms accumulating in oral malodor, essential oils have been included in mouthwashes [38], particularly mint oils inhibiting pathogens in the respiratory tract [38, 39]; essential oils also have beneficial organoleptic properties. Oral care preparations containing essential oils were found to be effective against oral malodor [40] with comparable activity to chlorhexidine [41]. Essential oils of anise, fennel, basil, and juniper berry in mouthwash, toothpaste, and mouth spray preparations were used to neutralize garlic odor in breath [42]. Lemongrass oil was shown as one of the efficient essential oils against *P. gingivalis* and was developed into an anti-oral pathogens mouthrinse (1%) with MIC and MBC of 0.0625 and 0.125 ppm, respectively. Although the lemongrass oil mouthrinse successfully suppressed oral malodor in clinical evaluated, it was not significant sensed by panelists [43]. A combination of the aroma compounds thymol, eucalyptol, menthol, and methyl salicylate from essential oils afforded anti-septic and anti-caries activities in dentifrices [44]. In addition, spearmint, peppermint, and eucalyptus oils were widely used for their therapeutic and psychological effects; tea tree oil was used to suppress oral malodor with methyl acetate and methyl lactate as anti-bacterial enhancers [45]. Furthermore, bay, bergamot, caraway, cedar, cinnamon, citronella, clove, coriander, laurel, lavender, lemon, marjoram, mustard, orange, orris, parley, pimento, pine, rosemary, sage, sassafras, terpentine, thyme, and witch hazel oils have been used in several dosage forms to reduce oral malodor [13, 39, 46].

Aroma compounds in essential oils have also been used in innovative products, such as complex compounds of menthol and anethole with β-cyclodextrin in lipsticks for breath refreshing [47]. In addition, the novel and efficient concept of treating bad breath with enzymes – i.e. protease, papain, bromelain, hydroxyalkyl cellulase, lipase, and glycoamylase – in order to remove tongue coating and further bacterial reduces is widely applied in different commercialized products.

6.4 ODOR MASKING FOR UNSCENTED/ ODORLESS/FRAGRANCE FREE PRODUCTS

In addition to a preference for pleasantly scented cosmetics, consumers tend to pay more attention to unscented/odorless/fragrance free products. The term 'fragrance free' straightforward depends on preparation without perfume/ fragrance/flavor additions; these unscented or odorless products are those without smells of their own. Accordingly, phytocosmetic actives with a pleasant smell are incorporated as a multifunctional ingredient. However, the key success is how to blend the phytocosmetic ingredients at the proper ratio to let them actively function as expected, while also perfuming/flavoring the product. For unscented/odorless products, the ingredients used should not be volatized or must be odorless. Advanced encapsulation technique and delivery system could be a successful solution; however, this choice will be more costly and threaten economic feasibility. Generally, additional masking agents are added to suppress the odor of the preparation. Cyclodextrins are the most common and cost effective ingredient for this task. Alternatively, starches, celluloses, and proteins derived from plants are also available for polymeric wall construction.

6.5 CONCLUSION

Several phytocosmetic sources offer a promising strategy to treat malodor. It should be noted that a mixture of the ingredients is found more commonly than the application of any single one. Furthermore, phytocosmetic ingredients are used in several forms – extracts (including essential and fix oils) or the isolated pure compounds. In particular, plant enzymes are preferred. A suitable delivery system/encapsulation technology to ensure efficacy of the phytocosmetics is a challenge. Phytocosmetics combating malodor are most obvious in commercialized toothpastes, as summarized in Table 6.1.

TABLE 6.1   Phytocosmetics for malodorant treatment

NAME		BENEFITS	
SCIENTIFIC	COMMON	BODY	ORAL
Abies cilicica	Cilician fir	✓	
Acacia catechu	Catechu		✓
Allium sativum	Garlic	✓	
Artocarpus spp.	-		✓
Calendula officinalis	Marigold	✓	
Camellia sinensis	Tea	✓	✓
Chaenomeles speciosa	Flowering quince	✓	
Commiphora myrrha	African myrrh	✓	
Corriandrum sativum	Coriander	✓	
Cuminum cyminum	Cumin	✓	
Daucus carota	Carrot	✓	
Echinophoria tenuifoli	Pickling herb	✓	
Foeniculum vulgare	Sweet fennel	✓	✓
Gaultheria procumbens	Wintergreen		✓
Ginkgo biloba	Gingko	✓	✓
Glycyrrhiza spp.	Licorice	✓	✓
Gunnera perpensa	Wild rhubarb	✓	
Harungana madagascariensis	Dragon's blood tree	✓	
Hibiscus sabdariffa	Roselle	✓	
Humulus lupulus	Hop	✓	✓
Malva sylvestris	Common mallow	✓	
Melaceuca alternifolia	Tea tree	✓	
Mentha spp.	Mint	✓	✓
Murraya paniculata	Orange jasmine		✓
Origanum spp.	Oregano/marjoram	✓	
Phellodendron amurense	Amur cork tree	✓	
Prunus armeniaca	Apricot	✓	
Rosmarinus officinalis	Rosemary	✓	
Salvia spp.	Sage	✓	✓

TABLE 6.1 (*Continued*)

NAME		BENEFITS	
SCIENTIFIC	COMMON	BODY	ORAL
Satureja spp.	Savoury	✓	
Sideritis spp.	Mountain tea	✓	
Simmodonsia chinensis	Jojoba	✓	
Smyrniopsis aucheri	-	✓	
Tamarix ramosissima	Salt cedar	✓	
Terminalia spp.	Terminalia	✓	✓
Thymbra spicata	Black thyme	✓	
Thymus sinenesi	Thyme	✓	
Vitis viticola	Grapevine downy mildew	✓	
Ziziphora spp.	Wild basil	✓	

Phytocosmetic ingredients

EXTRACT	ACTIVE
Aloe barbadensis, *Azadirachta indica* oil, caryophyllus oil, cinnamon, chamomile, *Clinacanthus nutans*, clove oil, *Emblica officinalis*, eucalyptus oil, fennel, *Foeniculum vulgare* oil, glycyrrhiza, grape fruit oil, guava, honey, licorice, *Mentha piperita* oil, nutmeg oil, *Ocimum basilicum* oil, orange jasmine, orange oil, para cress, peppermint oil, *Phyllanthus emblica*, sage, *Streblus asper*, *Terminalia bellerica*, *T. chebula*, toothbrush tree, wintergreen oil	Anisyl acetate, anise alcohol, anise aldehyde, benzaldehyde, benzyl alcohol, β-pinene, borneol, bromelain, camphor, caryophyllene alcohol, cinnamic aldehyde, dihydroeugenol, dihydrofarnesol, d-limonene, ethyl butyrate, ethyl octanoate, ethyl decanoate, farnesol, γ-decalactone, γ-terpinene, γ-undecalactone, hexyl alcohol, hexyl aldehyde, hinokitiol, isoeugenol, menthol, o-methoxycinnamic aldehyde, terpinolene, vitamin C, papain, protease

REFERENCES

1. Kanlayavattanakul M, Lourith N. Body malodours and their topical treatment agents. Int J Cosmet Sci. 2011;33:298–311.
2. Lourith N, Kanlayavattanakul M. Oral malodor and active ingredients for treatment. Int J Cosmet Sci. 2010;32: 321–9.
3. Cushine TPT, Lamb AJ. Antimicrobial activity of flavonoids. Int J Antimicrob Agents. 2005;26:343–56.

4. Higaki S, Morohashi M, Yamagishi T. Anti-lipase activity of Unsei-in against *Propionibacterium avidum* in the human axilla. Int J Antimicrob Agents. 2003;21:597–9.
5. Wecksser S, Engel K, Simon-Haarhaus B, et al. Screening of plant extracts for antimicrobial activity against bacteria and yeasts with dermatological relevance. Phytomedicine. 2007;14:508–16.
6. Baydar H, Sağdiç O, Özkan G, et al. Antibacterial activity and composition of essential oils from *Origanum*, *Thymbra* and *Satureja* spicies with commercial importance in Turkey. Food Control. 2004;15:169–72.
7. Özkan G, Sağdıç O, Özcan M. Inhibition of pathogenic bacteria by essential oils at different concentrations. Food Sci Technol Int. 2003;9:85–8.
8. Ebrahimi SN, Hadian J, Mirjalili MH, et al. Essential oil composition and antibacterial activity of *Thymus caramanicus* at different phenological stages. Food Chem. 2008;110:927–31.
9. Dayisoylu KS, Duman AD, Alma MH, et al. Antimicrobial activity of the essential oils of rosin from cones of *Abies cilicica* subsp. *cilicica*. Afr J Biotechnol. 2009;8:5021–4.
10. Arora DS, Kaur J. Antimicrobial activity of spices. Int J Antimicrob Agents. 1999;12:257–62.
11. Magee AR, van Wyk BE, van Vuuren SF. Ethnobotany and antimicrobial activity of sieketroos (Arctopus species). South Afr J Bot. 2007;73:159–62.
12. Yam TS, Shah S, Hamilton-Miller JMT. Microbiological activity of whole and fractioned crude extracts of tea (*Camellia sinensis*) and of tea components. FEMS Microbiol Lett. 1997;152:169–74.
13. Stier RE. Oral care compositions comprising diglycerol. US patent 6 723 304 B2. New Jersey: Noville Inc.; 2004.
14. Xianfei X, Xiaoqiang C, Shunying Z, et al. Chemical composition and antimicrobial activity of essential oils of *Chaenomeles speciosa* from China. Food Chem. 2007;100:1312–5.
15. Chappell KC, Scheeler PA, Rittershaus G. Herbal deodorant. US patent 5 256 405. Tom's of Maine: Maine; 1993.
16. Drewes SE, Khan F, van Vuuren SF, et al. Simple 1,4-benzoquinones with antibacterial activity from stems and leaves of *Gunnera perpensa*. Phytochemicine. 2005;66:1812–6.
17. Ueda M, Tokimitsu I, Masatoshi A. Deodorant for axillary odor. EU patent 0 433 911 A1. Kao Corp.: Tokyo; 1990.
18. Okoli AS, Okeke MI, Iroegbu CU, et al. Antibacterial activity of *Harungana madagascariensis* leaf extracts. Phytother Res. 2002;16:174–9.
19. Moulari B, Pellequer Y, Lboutounne H, et al. Isolation and in vitro antibacterial activity of astilbin, the bioactive flavanone from the leaves of *Harungana madagascariensis* Lam. Ex Poir. (Hypericaceae). J Ethnopharmacol. 2006;106:272–8.
20. Bockmuhl D, Hohne HM, Jassoy C, et al. Substances with a probiotic action used in deodorants. US patent 0 190 004 A1. Paul & Paul: Pennsylvania; 2007.
21. Dumas ER, Michaud AE, Bergeron C, et al. Deodorant effects of a supercritical hops extract: antibacterial activity against *Corynebacterium xerosis* and *Staphylococcus epidermidis* and efficacy testing of a hops/zinc ricinoleate stick in human through the sensory evaluation of axillary deodorancy. J Cosmet Dermatol. 2009;8:197–204.

22. Hammer KA, Carson CF, Riley TV. Susceptibility of transient and commensal skin flora to the essential oil of *Melaleuca alternifolia* (tea tree oil). Am J Infect Control. 1996;24:186–9.
23. Mikoshiba S, Takenaka H, Okumura T, et al. The suppressive effect of apricot kernel extract on 5α-androst-16-en-3-one generated by microbial metabolism. Int J Cosmet Sci. 2006;28:45–52.
24. Köse EO, Deniz İG, Sarıkürkçü C, et al. Chemical composition, antimicrobial and antioxidant activities of the essential oils of *Sideritis erythrantha* Boiss. and Heldr. (var. *erythrantha* and var. *cedretorum* P.H. Davis) endemic in Turkey. Food Chem Toxicol. 2010;48:2960–5.
25. Faridi P, Ghasemi Y, Gholami A, et al. Antimicrobial essential oil from *Smyrniopsis aucheri*. Chem Nat Com. 2008;44:116–8.
26. Vagionas K, Graikou K, Ngassapa O, et al. Composition and antimicrobial activity of the essential oils of three *Satureja* species growing in Tanzania. Food Chem. 2007;103:319–24.
27. Sultanova N, Makhmoor T, Abilov ZA, et al. Antioxidant and antimicrobial activities of *Tamarix ramosissima*. J Ethnopharmacol. 2001;78:201–5.
28. McManus K, Wood A, Wright MH, et al. *Terminalia ferdinandiana* Excell. extracts inhibit the growth of body odour-forming bacteria. Int J Cosmet Sci. 2017;39:500–10.
29. Cock IE, Wright MH, Matthews B, et al. Bioactive compounds sourced from *Terminalia* spp. in bacterial malodour prevention: an effective alternative to chemical additives. Int J Cosmet Sci. 2019;41:496–508.
30. Ozturk S, Ercisli S. Antibacterial activity and chemical constitutions of *Ziziphora clinopodioides*. Food Control. 2007;18:535–40.
31. Ozturk S, Ercisli S. The chemical composition of essential oil and *in vitro* antibacterial activities of essential oil and methanol extract of *Ziziphora persica* Bunge. J Ethnopharmacol. 2006;106:372–6.
32. Akiba S, Ara K, Kusuoku H, et al. Deodorant agent. US patent 0 251 296 A1. Kao Corp.: Tokyo; 2006.
33. Wang CK, Chen SL, Wu MG. Inhibitory effect of betel quid on the volatility of methyl mercaptan. J Agric Food Chem. 2001;49:1979–83.
34. Ramji N, Ramji N, Iyer R, et al. Phenolic antibacterials from *Piper betel* in the prevention of haliotosis. J Ethnopharmacol. 2002;83:149–52.
35. Zhou JH. Composition and method for inhibiting oral bacteria. US patent 6 319 523 B1. Cincinnati; 2001.
36. Garlich JR, Masterson TT, Frank RK. Phytate antimicrobial compounds in oral care products. US patent 5 300 289. Michigan: Dow Chemical Co.; 1994.
37. Sterer N, Nuas S, Mizrahi B, et al. Oral malodor reduction by a palatal mucoadhesive tablet containing herbal formulation. J Dent. 2008;36:535–9.
38. Edris AE. Pharmaceutical and therapeutic potentials of essential oils and their individual volatile constituents: a review. Phytotherapy Res. 2007;21: 308–23.
39. Tashjian A, Mills S. Hygiene mouthspray composition. US patent 6 579 513 B1. Cincinnati: Playtex Products Inc.; 2003.
40. Olshan AM, Kohut BE, Vincent JW, et al. Clinical effectiveness of essential oil-containing dentifrices in controlling oral malodor. Am J Dent. 2000;13:18C–22C.

41. Charles C, Mostler K, Bartels L, et al. Comparative antiplaque and antigingivitis effectiveness of a chlorhexidine and an essential oil mouthrinse: 6 months clinical trial. J Clin Periodontol. 2004;31:878–4.
42. Pilch S, Williams M, Vazquez J. Oral care malodor composition. US patent 0 134 023 A1. New Jersey: Colgate-Palmolive Co.; 2006.
43. Satthanakul P, Taweechaisupapong S, Paphangkorakit J, et al. Antimicrobial effect of lemongrass oil against oral malodour micro-organisms and the pilot study of safety and efficacy of lemongrass mouthrinse on oral malodour. J App Microbiol. 2014;118:11–7.
44. Harper DS, Parikh RM, Alli D, et al. Antiseptic dentifrice. US patent 5 942 211. New Jersey: Warner-Lambert Co.; 1999.
45. Liu X, Williams M, Subramanyam R, et al. Oral composition for reducing mouth odors. US patent 6 379 652 B1. New Jersey: Colgate-Palmolive Co.; 2002.
46. Pan P, Finnegan M, Soshinsky A, et al. Oral care compositions comprising tropolone compounds and essential oils and methods of using the same. US patent 6 689 342 B1. New Jersey: Warner-Lambert Co.; 2004.
47. Meyers AJ, Lutrario CA, Elliott M, et al. Breath freshening lipstick. US patent 6 383 475 B1. Delaware: FD Management Inc.; 2002.

Phytocosmetics Delivery Technology

7

Henry H.Y. Tong and Aviva S.F. Chow

Contents

7.1 INTRODUCTION

With increasing consumer expectations, greater product differentiation pressure, tighter cost control, and higher concerns in efficacy and safety, cosmetic scientists are facing many challenges in their professional practices. The optimal delivery of cosmetic actives should be sought to secure sustainable beauty effects, enhancing consumer experiences and brand loyalty therein. In cosmetic product development, it is not uncommon for marketing professionals to make decision in the choice of cosmetic actives and the associated potential claims for the products first. The formulators then need to materialize the concept in their laboratory, pondering what to do with the given assignment and how to wrap it up as an elegant cosmetic product for the coming presentation. Unfortunately, the timeline is usually short, as a downstream stability test and user test will be needed for a further push from idea to market. In today's fast-paced world, a quick return on R&D investment is always necessary.

With the advancement of cosmetic technology, formulation experts are now armed with a plethora of generic and patented delivery platforms to address the aforementioned challenges. Yet the ultimate question still remains in the many formulators' minds: Which delivery technology should I use for my current project and the chosen cosmetic active?

In this chapter, the question is addressed by using a hypothetical example of the phytocosmetic active "resveratrol". Self-reflection is used for the imaginary journey in formulating resveratrol as a cosmetic product. Instead of reviewing each delivery method in a standalone format, it is sincerely wished that this will be a starting point for better formulation strategy among our readers.

7.2 KNOW YOUR COMPOUND FIRST

Resveratrol (Figure 7.1A) was first isolated in *Vitis vinifera* (the common grape vine). It is reported to exert anti-oxidation effects, UV photoprotection and skin anti-aging effects [1], tyrosinase inhibition, anti-melanogenesis and skin lightening effects [2], and collagen production stimulation and anti-inflammatory effects, *Propionicbacterium acne* inhibition and anti-acne effects [3]. The usage of topical preparation with 1% resveratrol, 0.5% baicalin, and 1% vitamin E shows statistically improvement in fine lines, wrinkles, skin firmness, skin elasticity, skin laxity, hyperpigmentation, radiation, and skin roughness

(A)

(B)

	Micellar system	Vesicular system	Particulate systems
Representative formulations	Microemulsion; Nanoemulsion	Liposome; Niosome	Micro-particle suspension; Nano-particle suspension
Commercial examples in resveratrol	African Botanics Cloudburst Microemulsion Balancing Moisturizer	Resveraderm Liposomal Serum; Renue Transdermal Lotion with Liposomal NAD+	Sephora The Ordinary 3% resveratrol + 3% ferulic acid
Advantages to be used in cosmetics	Easy for scale-up & manufacture; Cost-effective in large-scale production; Excellent physical stability if properly formulated	Excellent skin compatibility; Enhanced dermal delivery of phytocosmetic with minimal skin irritation	Particle engineering possible for specific delivery, such as follicular delivery; Solid deposition on skin surface for sustained release of phytocosmetics
Disadvantages to be used in cosmetics	Relatively time-consuming during R&D process; Precipitation upon dilution can be a concern	Retention of liposomal structure in final finished dosage form can be challenging	Long-term stability, particularly for physical stability, can be challenging, and needs careful optimization

(C)

	Principle	Application in cosmetics
Rheology measurement	Torque is measured upon variation of spindle speeds, resulting in stress/shear rate curve, and viscosity profile	Viscosity measurement is very important in cosmetics, as it is closely linked with many parameters in consumer experiences, such as rub-in, firmness.
Texture profile analysis	Force is measured upon variation in probe displacement, resulting in force/time & force/distance curves	Texture profile analysis yields good match with some parameters in consumer experiences, such as friction, spreadability
Microscopic analysis	Many techniques are available in this category, including optical microscopy, scanning electron microscopy	Evaluation of cosmetics micro-environment is possible, particularly important for advanced delivery systems
Thermal analysis	Differential scanning calorimetry allows heat flow measurement against temperature under programmed scanning, and performs best if coupled with thermogravimetric analysis	Thermal behavior of cosmetic can be revealed, such as glass transition temperature, melting endotherm, dehydration temperature.
Particle size analysis	Many techniques are available in this category, including analytical sieving, microscopic evaluation, coulter counter, and laser diffraction	Particle size distribution evaluation is important in assessing long-term stability of cosmetics; Consumer experiences are compromised if particle size control is poor

FIGURE 7.1 (A) Resveratrol, (B) Micellar, vesicular, and particulate systems in resveratrol, and (C) Commonly used physical characterization methods in cosmetics development.

over baseline [4]. Resveratrol gel (0.009% w/w) results in 53.75% mean reduction in the Global Acne Grading System score [5]. Resveratrol (0.01% w/w) in a w/o cream shows visible signs of clinical improvement in terms of skin parameters such as corneometry, elastometry, and colorimetry [6].

Resveratrol is well established in that solute lipophilicity and skin penetration are highly related [7]. Resveratrol has an excellent safety profile [8] with facial redness reducing ability [9]. A good choice of delivery method will not only allow optimal target site delivery in skin, allowing beauty effects, but will also enable less usage of expensive phytocosmetics for the same biological effects, decreasing the unit cost.

7.3 SIMPLICITY IS THE BEST

The advantages of traditional dosage forms of cosmetics as delivery methods are a simple formula, great in cost control, good availability in most cosmetic manufacturers, and most importantly, good consumer acceptability. As a result, most cosmetic products in the market belong to this category of delivery methods. There are many formulation strategies available in traditional cosmetic dosage forms to enhance phytocosmetic delivery. Optimizing vehicle pH value is a common option. The acidic dissociation constants in resveratrol are determined to be: $pK_{a1} = 8.01$, $pK_{a2} = 9.86$, and $pK_{a3} = 10.50$. The lower pH values would result in non-ionized forms, theoretically enhancing passive diffusion across stratum corneum. It is reported that in an *in-vitro* Franz diffusion cell experiment, resveratrol calibrated skin disposition (drug amount in skin/solubility) at pH 6, 8, 9.9, and 10.8 are 303.03, 273.62, 17.37, and 5.85 $\mu g/g$, respectively [10].

Vehicle manipulation is another common option for enhancing skin absorption of phytocosmetics. When pomegranate seed oil is increased from 2.5%, 5.0% to 10.0%, the permeation co-efficients of resveratrol across pig skin are increased from 1.63, 2.87 to 4.67×10^{-2} cm/h [11]. It has been reported that increasing oil content in an o/w cream from 25/75 to 50/50 results in significant decreases in initial release co-efficients, diffusion co-efficients within the formulation, and skin permeation co-efficients for resveratrol. It is speculated that the hydrophobic resveratrol is located inside the oil-phase, with the need to overcome the interface oil/water prior to the diffusion across pig skin in Franz diffusion experiment [12].

Although resveratrol can penetrate into skin by traditional delivery methods, cosmetokinetic data alone are not sufficient and should be verified by cosmetodynamic-cosmetokinetic relationship. Upon application of a resveratrol dose of 409.88 nmol/cm^2 across pig skin, 375.26 nmol/cm^2 stays on the surface, with skin penetration into stratum corneum, epidermis, and dermis at 13.71, 2.02, and 0.39 nmol/cm^2 [13]. An anti-oxidative effect for resveratrol, measured by the free radical 1,1'-diphenyl-2-picrylhydrazyl scavenging test (DPPH test), is observed in the stratum corneum, epidermis, and dermis at 1.7, 12.8, and 44.9 nmol/cm^2 in the samples [13, 14]. On first impression, this relationship does not make sense, as there should be positive correlation between resveratrol concentration and anti-oxidative effect, not negative correlation. The underlying reason is possibly due to skin metabolism of resveratrol. Upon skin application, it is reported that resveratrol can be converted into its glucuronized form, which are believed to retain pharmacological actions. Relative abundance differences of the metabolites are found in topical resveratrol via different vehicles – i.e., ethanol, hydrophilic ointment, macrogol gel, and carboxymethylcellulose gel – with water soluble gels – i.e., the latter two gel preparations – exhibiting the greatest efficiencies in trans-dermal resveratrol absorption and penetration [15].

7.4 WHEN SHOULD WE NOT BE SATISFIED WITH THE ROUTINES?

The usual concept of "the more skin absorption there is, the better a delivery method" does not apply to phytocosmetic delivery. This is because phytocosmetics are intended to provide a beauty effect confined to the skin layer. Phytocosmetic delivery should focus on a targeted site in skin delivery. Only if the outcomes – i.e., firm proof in beauty effects and lack of systemic and local side effects – are clearly defined, advanced delivery method would justify the additional cost needed.

Advanced delivery methods have three major categories: micellar systems (such as micro- and nano-emulsions), vesicular systems (such as liposomes and niosomes), and particulate systems (such as micro- and nano-particles based on polymers and/or lipids). Pros and cons are summarized in Figure 7.1B.

7.4.1 Micellar Systems

Micro-emulsion is a thermodynamically stable preparation composed of an aqueous phase, an oil phase, a surfactant, and a co-surfactant component, which can be summarized as a ternary phase diagram. During formulation exercise, formulators should find an optimal design space in phytocosmetic active solubilization, and more importantly, there should be a lack of precipitation and phase separation upon water dilution. Once the sweet spot is found, micro-emulsion can enable high solubilization capacity for both hydrophilic and lipophilic cosmetic actives. Micro-emulsion manufacturing is straightforward, as simple mixing tanks would be good enough for the purpose. A novel oil-in-water (o/w)-type micro-emulsion, utilizing sucrose laurate, isopropyl myristate/ethanol, and water as the components, has been examined in Yucatan micro-pig skin. Delivery of resveratrol was achieved, and enabled by albumin binding [16]. Replacing sucrose laurate with sucrose oleate in the micro-emulsion formulation results in a 5× fold increase in skin penetration [17]. Therefore, the micro-emulsion formulation approach is an option in resveratrol dermal delivery for sustainable effects. Although the beauty effect is now enhanced, care should be taken to observe any potential side effects in skin, as resveratrol will now remain in skin for a much longer period of time.

Compared with thermodynamically stable micro-emulsion, nano-emulsion is a thermodynamically unstable micellar system that is kinetically stabilized with a low surfactant/co-surfactant concentration, i.e., usually smaller than <10% w/v. High energy methods, such as micro-fluidization or sonication, are used during the manufacturing process. Clearly, physical stability of micro-emulsion is better than that of nano-emulsion; however, topical application of nano-emulsion is highly likely to be more skin-friendly, as the concentration of irritant surfactant can be reduced to a bare minimum, suitable for clients with sensitive skin. Yet scaling-up can be a problem for nano-emulsion, as micro-fluidization or sonication are not common as equipment available in the cosmetic industry. Theranostic resveratrol nano-emulsion has been used to map skin biodistribution after topical application. Interestingly, it has been shown that the preparation is non-toxic at doses of up to 20 μM, readily internalized by macrophages *in vitro*, and significantly lowers the nitric oxide generation in lipopolysaccharide-activated macrophages *in vitro*, without causing cell viability changes [18]. The finding is interesting to cosmetic scientists, as the data are highly relevant to the beauty claims in detoxification and anti-pollution. Resveratrol nano-emulsion may be positioned in a high-end market, with the high cost associated with manufacturing, but care should be taken in translating the positive *in-vitro* data in resveratrol skin delivery into real *in-vivo* beauty effects.

Surfactants are the most important components in micelle formation within micellar systems. In order to further improve targeted site delivery of phytocosmetics, polymers with surfactant property have been utilized to form a micellar system. Polyethylene glycol (PEG)–poly(gamma-benzyl-L-glutamate) (PBLG) copolymer has been chosen to form polymeric micelles in resveratrol, enabling an active ingredient with preferential staying in the living cell layer of stratum corneum [19]. This would have a theoretical advantage in minimizing skin side effects, but further clinical data are still needed to justify the advantages noted in *in-vitro* studies.

7.4.2 Vesicular Systems

Liposomes, with a lipid bilayer, are able to encapsulate hydrophobic drugs and cosmetic actives in their lipophilic core, assisting the chemical of interest to pass through cell membranes. In topical delivery, liposomes are well known to have good encapsulation of cosmetic actives for effective delivery and clinical proven beauty effects. When resveratrol is incorporated within a standard soybean phosphatidylcholine lipid bilayer liposomal structure, resveratrol is located near the phosphocholine head groups, which are able to solubilize it to a 150 × increase of aqueous solubility in water, with easy diffusion through liposomal membranes [20]. Resveratrol has also been wrapped in topical liposomal formulation via mixing resveratrol with ethoxydiglycol, followed by homogenization with Pentravan® vehicle. The skin absorption of resveratrol is effective with a relative bioavailability of 62.65% via skin route [21]. Comparatively speaking, a topical ethanolic solution of resveratrol, with a total dose of 409.88 nmol/cm² applied on porcine skin, only results in 3.34%, 0.49%, 0.09% and undetectable disposition of in stratum corneum, epidermis, dermis, and receptor fluid, respectively [13]. Besides standard liposome structures, it is possible to make use of the versatility of liposomal structures by including functional components in these vesicular systems. Penetration enhancers, such as caprylyl/capryl polyglucosides and propylene glycol monolaurate, have been included in resveratrol liposomes, enabling deep embedding of resveratrol within the bilayer structure [22]. In addition, deformability of liposome can be engineered by including soy phosphatidylcholine, Tween 80, and cholesterol, with fluidity enhancement of the liposome bilayers in the region of the phospholipid hydrophobic chains, facilitating resveratrol accommodation within the bilayer [23]. The skin absorption of liposomal resveratrol is so good that it is possible for this dietary supplement to be administered by the topical route in liposomal formulation, rather than oral intake. Should liposomal resveratrol be able to have mass production, the great enhancement of its skin bioavailability can have good cost control, as the phytocosmetic dose needed would be much reduced by this enhanced delivery method.

Since the success is attested for liposomes, there are many modified versions of liposome and vesicular systems. Niosomes, for example, are similar to liposomes, with significant improvement in compatibility, stability, and toxicity. The major difference between liposomes and niosomes is that nonionic surfactant is utilized in niosomes. Resveratrol-loaded niosome has been prepared by Tween 60 in water, resulting in vesicular system with 471–565 nm hydrodynamic diameter, good *in vitro* permeation behavior, and good anti-oxidation properties [24]. In another study, resveratrol-loaded niosome was made by a surfactant – i.e., Gelot 64 – and two penetration enhancers with great skin compatibility – i.e., oleic acid and linoleic acid [25]. Compared with resveratrol-loaded liposome, resveratrol-loaded niosome has similar average size (~180–220 nm), polydispersity index, entrapment efficiency, and defor-mation index, but much higher stratum corneum distribution and much more *ex-vivo* diffusion of vesicular resveratrol through newborn pig skin [26]. Resveratrol-loaded niosome from Span 80 and cholesterol, after incorporation into a Carbopol 934 gel at 1% w/w level as an bio-adhesive vehicle, was found to have much better and faster pharmacokinetic parameters in stratum cor-neum (2.07 × time increase in AUC_{-0-6h}; 2.05 × time increase in C_{max}; 0.55 time decrease in T_{max}), compared with resveratrol-loaded suspension [27]. Since non-ionic surfactants are well known to have fewer topical side effects than cat-ionic and anionic surfactants, niosomes can be a good alternative to liposomes.

Besides liposomes and niosomes, there are many modifications of vesicular systems, resulting in a wide range of "-osome" technology. Examples include ethosome, glycerosome, trans-ferosome, and phytosome. Ethosome is charac-terized by a high content of ethanol and is regarded as an acceptable co-solvent in cosmetic product. Resveratrol-loaded ethosome is loaded in 1% Carbopol 934P gel, resulting in 62.75–64.60% skin retention of resveratrol, compared with 6.80% for resveratrol in ethanol solution and 14.05% for resveratrol in cream base [28]. On top of enhanced delivery in resveratrol, ethosome is defi-nitely suitable for usage in toners and astringents, with the capability of giving a cooling sensation due to its high ethanol content. Glycerosome, which con-tains glycerol at 50% v/v or more, is obviously suitable in phytocosmetic deliv-ery, as glycerol is one of the most commonly used natural moisturizing factors for skin hydration. Glycerol for vesicular system construction can change the dielectric constant in an inter-vesicle medium and the subsequent orientation of the phospholipid chain; resveratrol-loaded glycerosomes from Poloxamer and glycerol has therefore been prepared for bio-protection on inflamed skin. It is reported that the vesicles are spherical, unilamellar, and small in size – i.e., ~70 nm in diameter – and most importantly, able to protect fibroblasts from chemical-induced oxidative damage and reduce oedema and leukocyte infil-tration on phorbol ester exposed skin. Trans-ferosome is equipped with the introduction of non-ionic edge activators, enhancing the flexibility and deform-ability of vesicular structures, compared with liposome. This allows easy pen-etration through skin pores much smaller than itself and dermal penetration with sustained release of active components. Using Tween 20, Plantacare® 1200 UP, and Tween 80 as non-ionic edge activators, resveratrol-loaded trans-ferosome is reported to improve instability, solubility, bioavailability, and safety of resveratrol [29]. Another study utilizing Tween 80 to produce resveratrol-loaded trans-ferosome shows similar advantages, with better cytoxicity demonstrated in a number of *in-vitro* safety studies [30]. Phytosome, as the name suggests, is the liposome derived from natural-based materials, with concepts similar to phytocosmetics. Resveratrol-loaded phytosome, composed of phosphatidylcholine and incorporated into a transdermal patch, is reported to have sustainable therapeutic effects in treating acute and chronic inflammation [31].

The evolution of vesicular systems clearly demonstrates three points: (1) In view of a wide diversity of vesicular systems, formulators should focus on not only the delivery method but also the presentation of finished dosage form, as different vesicle systems are obviously more suitable for different kinds of final presentations. (2) A phytodelivery method of phytocosmetic is totally possible for enhanced delivery, without usage of any synthetic materials in the process, although the quality uniformity of natural-based products is still a concern. (3) Many cosmetic ingredient suppliers are now providing intermediates, such as liposomes and niosomes. Formulators need to consider whether the vesicular systems are still stable in the designed vehicle. The question would be technically challenging if many other cosmetic actives are already included. Yet, quality control in the finished dosage form is usually not easy in vesicular systems. Although the availability of many vesicular forms gives formulators extra freedom in formulation, it also results in extra uncertainties in these chemically complex systems.

7.4.3 Particulate Systems

The major differences between particulate systems and vesicular systems are the presence of solid phase materials in the former. The solid materials can be micro-sized, i.e., micro-particles, or nano-sized, i.e., nano-particles and nano-structured materials. In this category of cosmetic products, although the cost of production would be higher than traditional dosage forms, large scale manufacturing under mass production is possible, as particle engineering is becoming a mature technology.

Solid lipid micro-particles, popular as a skin-friendly material, have been much utilized to encapsulate cosmetic actives, including resveratrol. Resveratrol solid lipid micro-particles, prepared by melt dispersion technique without the use of any organic solvents, are able to produce resveratrol in an amorphous state, allowing rapid dissolution and bioactivity [32]. Resveratrol-loaded solid lipid micro-particles, if coated with chitosan, can further enhance skin penetration of resveratrol [33]. In the modern cosmetic supply chain, micro-particles of popular cosmeceuticals, such as resveratrol, are expected to be commercially available. Formulators can readily refer to the in-house technical dossier for physicochemical properties, biological effects, and clinical evidence of the micro-particles involved. It should particularly be noted that the biological properties cannot be cross-referenced across intermediates from different brand names, as micro-particles formulation is highly material- and process-dependent.

Resveratrol nano-suspension, obtained by wet milling and suspended in 1–2% of surfactants P188 or T80, is reported to result in better skin penetration and higher dermal anti-oxidant properties in the skin layer [34]. Resveratrol-loaded composite nano-particles produced by supercritical fluid crystallization have been found to enhance *in-vitro* permeation of resveratrol [35]. In resveratrol-loaded chitosan/gum Arabic nano-particles using the Pickering emulsion system, skin retention of resveratrol is increased with good photostability in resveratrol [36]. Resveratrol nano-capsules, with grape seed oil as core and poly(ε-caprolactone) as polymeric shell, are reported to have interaction with human dermal fibroblasts [37]. Nano-structured carriers of resveratrol are minimal in skin toxicity [38]. However, resveratrol-loaded nano-particles are found to have much lower IC_{50} in a number of *in-vitro* cytotoxicity studies [39]. The higher toxicity indicated is a great deterrent for formulators. High skin retention of the phytocosmetic, with no systemic bioavailability, is strictly required in cosmetic industry. Additionally, nano-particles always have a problem with long-term stability, as the high surface area of solids renders the preparation highly unstable. The intrinsic high physical instability is usually overcome by incorporation with lots of surfactants to avoid particle agglomeration, but high surfactant concentration can damage the skin barrier function. In view of increasing health concerns, high costs of materials, and the challenging formulation exercise for stabilization, it may be wise to avoid nano-sized phytocosmetics unless the safety data are scientifically convincing enough for their usage in cosmetic products.

For advanced delivery of phytocosmetics, the physical characterization summarized in Figure 7.1C is important during formulation development to ensure efficacy, quality, and safety for consumer uses.

7.5 FUTURE PROSPECTS OF PHYTOCOSMETICS DELIVERY

There is a need for formulators to develop delivery platforms, with well-researched design space, allowing variations in cosmetic actives and other ingredients at pre-specified ranges. An increasing number of formulation exercises in phytocosmetics delivery should be dedicated to skincare personalization in the future.

The phytocosmetic delivery system developed by formulators needs not only to address clients' sophisticated beauty needs but also to remain physically, chemically, and microbiologically stable under different environmental challenges, including a supply chain across different geographic regions and global warming. An increasing number of formulation exercises in phytocosmetics delivery should be dedicated to stability enhancement in the future.

7.6 CONCLUSION

This chapter provides a brief overview in delivery technologies available for cosmetic formulators, using phytocosmetic resveratrol as an illustration. Advanced delivery methods, such as micellar system, vesicular system and particulate systems, are covered. Future prospects in phytocosmetics delivery are also mentioned, though there is much more for formulators to learn, as all of us will be witnessing fast advancement of cosmetic science and technology in the coming future.

REFERENCES

1. Chedea VS, Vicaş SI, Sticozzi C, et al. Resveratrol: from diet to topical usage. Food Funct. 2017;8(11):3879–92.
2. Boo YC. Human skin lightening efficacy of resveratrol and its analogs: from in vitro studies to cosmetic applications. Antioxidants (Basel). 2019;8(9):332.
3. Ratz-Łyko A, Arct J. Resveratrol as an active ingredient for cosmetic and dermatological applications: a review. J Cosmet Laser Ther. 2019;21(2):84–90.
4. Farris P, Yatskayer M, Chen N, et al. Evaluation of efficacy and tolerance of a nighttime topical antioxidant containing resveratrol, baicalin, and vitamin e for treatment of mild to moderately photodamaged skin. J Drugs Dermatol. 2014;13(12):1467–72.
5. Fabbrocini G, Staibano S, De Rosa G, et al. Resveratrol-containing gel for the treatment of acne vulgaris: a single-blind, vehicle-controlled, pilot study. Am J Clin Dermatol. 2011;12(2):133–41.
6. Moyano-Mendez JR, Fabbrocini G, De Stefano D, et al. Enhanced antioxidant effect of trans-resveratrol: potential of binary systems with polyethylene glycol and cyclodextrin. Drug Dev Ind Pharm. 2014;40(10):1300–7.

7. Cross SE, Magnusson BM, Winckle G, et al. Determination of the effect of lipophilicity on the *in vitro* permeability and tissue reservoir characteristics of topically applied solutes in human skin layers. J Invest Dermatol. 2003;120(5):759–64.

8. Fiume MM, Bergfeld WF, Belsito DV, et al. Safety assessment of *Vitis vinifera* (grape)-derived ingredients as used in cosmetics. Int J Toxicol. 2014;33(3 suppl):48s–83s.

9. Ferzli G, Patel M, Phrsai N, et al. Reduction of facial redness with resveratrol added to topical product containing green tea polyphenols and caffeine. J Drugs Dermatol. 2013;12(7):770–4.

10. Hung CF, Lin YK, Huang ZR, et al. Delivery of resveratrol, a red wine polyphenol, from solutions and hydrogels via the skin. Biol Pharm Bull. 2008;31(5):955–62.

11. Liu W, Zhao Q, Lv L, et al. Pomegranate seed oil enhances the percutaneous absorption of trans-resveratrol. J Oleo Sci. 2018;67(4):479–87.

12. Zillich OV, Schweiggert-Weisz U, Hasenkopf K, et al. Release and in vitro skin permeation of polyphenols from cosmetic emulsions. Int J Cosmet Sci. 2013;35(5):491–501.

13. Alonso C, Rubio L, Touriño S, et al. Antioxidative effects and percutaneous absorption of five polyphenols. Free Radic Biol Med. 2014;75:149–55.

14. Alonso C, Martí M, Barba C, et al. Skin permeation and antioxidant efficacy of topically applied resveratrol. Arch Dermatol Res. 2017;309(6):423–31.

15. Murakami I, Chaleckis R, Pluskal T, et al. Metabolism of skin-absorbed resveratrol into its glucuronized form in mouse skin. PLoS One. 2014;9(12):e115359.

16. Yutani R, Kikuchi T, Teraoka R, et al. Efficient delivery and distribution in skin of chlorogenic acid and resveratrol induced by microemulsion using sucrose laurate. Chem Pharm Bull (Tokyo). 2014;62(3):274–80.

17. Yutani R, Komori Y, Takeuchi A, et al. Prominent efficiency in skin delivery of resveratrol by novel sucrose oleate microemulsion. J Pharm Pharmacol. 2016;68(1):46–55.

18. Herneisey M, Williams J, Mirtic J, et al. Development and characterization of resveratrol nanoemulsions carrying dual-imaging agents. Ther Deliv. 2016;7(12):795–808.

19. Yotsumoto K, Ishii K, Kokubo M, et al. Improvement of the skin penetration of hydrophobic drugs by polymeric micelles. Int J Pharm. 2018;553(1-2):132–40.

20. Cardia MC, Caddeo C, Lai F, et al. 1H NMR study of the interaction of trans-resveratrol with soybean phosphatidylcholine liposomes. Sci Rep. 2019;9(1):17736.

21. Polonini HC, Bastos Cde A, de Oliveira MA, et al. *In vitro* drug release and *ex vivo* percutaneous absorption of resveratrol cream using HPLC with zirconized silica stationary phase. J Chromatogr B Analyt Technol Biomed Life Sci. 2014;947–948:23–31.

22. Caddeo C, Manconi M, Cardia MC, et al. Investigating the interactions of resveratrol with phospholipid vesicle bilayer and the skin: NMR studies and confocal imaging. Int J Pharm. 2015;484(1–2):138–45.

23. Tosato MG, Maya Girón J V, Martin A A, et al. Comparative study of transdermal drug delivery systems of resveratrol: high efficiency of deformable liposomes. Mater Sci Eng C Mater Biol Appl. 2018;90:356–64.

24. Tavano L, Muzzalupo R, Picci N, et al. Co-encapsulation of lipophilic antioxidants into niosomal carriers: percutaneous permeation studies for cosmeceutical applications. Colloids Surf B Biointerfaces. 2014;114:144–9.

25. Pando D, Matos M, Gutiérrez G, et al. Formulation of resveratrol entrapped niosomes for topical use. Colloids Surf B Biointerfaces. 2015;128:398–404.
26. Pando D, Caddeo C, Manconi M, et al. Nanodesign of olein vesicles for the topical delivery of the antioxidant resveratrol. J Pharm Pharmacol. 2013;65(8):1158–67.
27. Negi P, Aggarwal M, Sharma G, et al. Niosome-based hydrogel of resveratrol for topical applications: an effective therapy for pain related disorder(s). Biomed Pharmacother. 2017;88:480–7.
28. Arora D, Nanda S. Quality by design driven development of resveratrol loaded ethosomal hydrogel for improved dermatological benefits via enhanced skin permeation and retention. Int J Pharm. 2019;567:118448.
29. Caddeo C, Manca ML, Matos M, et al. Functional response of novel bioprotective poloxamer-structured vesicles on inflamed skin. Nanomedicine. 2017;13(3):1127–36.
30. Scognamiglio I, De Stefano D, Campani V, et al. Nanocarriers for topical administration of resveratrol: a comparative study. Int J Pharm. 2013;440(2):179–87.
31. Kalita B, Das MK, Sarma M, et al. Sustained anti-inflammatory effect of resveratrol-phospholipid complex embedded polymeric patch. AAPS Pharm Sci Tech. 2017;18(3):629–45.
32. Angellotti G, Murgia D, Presentato A, et al. Antibacterial PE gylated solid lipid microparticles for cosmeceutical purpose: formulation, characterization, and efficacy evaluation. Materials (Basel). 2020;13(9):1–17.
33. Scalia S, Trotta V, Iannuccelli V, et al. Enhancement of in vivo human skin penetration of resveratrol by chitosan-coated lipid microparticles. Colloids Surf B Biointerfaces. 2015;135:42–9.
34. Sinico C, Pireddu R, Pini E, et al. Enhancing topical delivery of resveratrol through a nanosizing approach. Planta Med. 2017;83(5):476–81.
35. Ha ES, Sim WY, Lee SK, et al. Preparation and evaluation of resveratrol-loaded composite nanoparticles using a supercritical fluid technology for enhanced oral and skin delivery. Antioxidants (Basel). 2019;8(11):1–17.
36. Sharkawy A, Casimiro FM, Barreiro MF, et al. Enhancing trans-resveratrol topical delivery and photostability through entrapment in chitosan/gum Arabic Pickering emulsions. Int J Biol Macromol. 2020;147:150–9.
37. Friedrich RB, Kann B, Coradini K, et al. Skin penetration behavior of lipid-core nanocapsules for simultaneous delivery of resveratrol and curcumin. Eur J Pharm Sci. 2015;78:204–13.
38. Tsai MJ, Lu IJ, Fu YS, et al. Nanocarriers enhance the transdermal bioavailability of resveratrol: *in-vitro* and *in-vivo* study. Colloids Surf B Biointerfaces. 2016;148:650–6.
39. Rocha V, Marques C, Figueiredo JL, et al. *In vitro* cytotoxicity evaluation of resveratrol-loaded nanoparticles: focus on the challenges of in vitro methodologies. Food Chem Toxicol. 2017;103:214–22.

Safety Assessment of Phytocosmetics

8

M. Pilar Vinardell

Contents

8.1 INTRODUCTION

Phytocosmetics have been used traditionally by many cultures. In recent years, there has been an increasing amount of interest among consumers for natural cosmetics as they are considered less toxic than the cosmetics containing synthetic chemicals. Nevertheless, natural cosmetics should be evaluated in the same way as synthetic cosmetics to demonstrate their safety (Figure 8.1A).

There is a popular misconception that being natural is equal to being safe, a myth supported by the media as well as political and economic stakeholders [1]. However, natural products can be toxic or have potential human health risks.

(A)

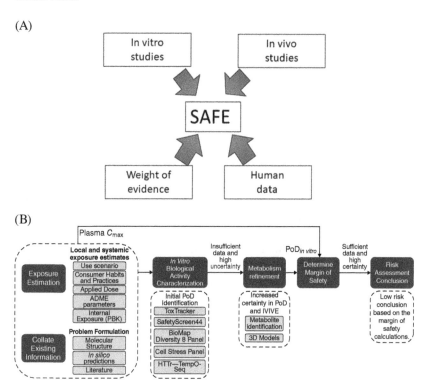

(B)

FIGURE 8.1 (A) Phytocosmetics, which are cosmetics with a botanical origin, should be safe for consumers based on *in vivo* and *in vitro* studies as well as human data and the weight of evidence. (B) Next generation risk assessment workflow for 0.1% coumarin in consumer products. HTTr, high-throughput transcriptomics; IVIVE, *in vitro* to *in vivo* extrapolation [55].

8.1.1 Regulations

In the European Union (EU), the European Cosmetic Directive 76/768/EC was introduced in 1976 and is periodically updated [2].

According to this regulation, cosmetics do not require pre-market clearance. It is the responsibility of the manufacturer to ensure the safety of the cosmetic products and their ingredients. However, certain ingredients require approval prior to marketing, such as colorants, hair dyes, preservatives, and UV filters. All of these are included in the respective annexes of the Directive. Banned ingredients are listed in Annex II of the Directive and include some substances that do not have enough data to support their safety. Concentration-limited substances are listed in Annex III of the Directive. In the EU, the approval process includes the submission of a safety dossier to the EU Scientific Committee on Consumer Safety (SCCS), which issues an opinion on the safety of the ingredient. Safety requirements for cosmetic ingredients are listed in the "Notes of Guidance for the Testing of Cosmetic Ingredients and their Safety Evaluation," which is updated periodically and represents a guideline for safety evaluations [3].

In Europe, the SCCS advises the European Commission about the safety of cosmetics through opinions of the different ingredients present in cosmetics. However, little attention has been paid to botanical ingredients and only a few of them have been evaluated by the SCCS.

In the EU, manufacturers and importers of cosmetic products are required to generate a safety dossier on each cosmetic product, which should include the composition, specifications and a product safety assessment of the final product as well as its ingredients. The safety assessment has to be performed by a qualified expert.

The United States (US) Food, Drug, and Cosmetic Act of 1938 designated the US Food and Drug Administration (FDA) as the agency responsible for the safety of cosmetics. The provisions of this act ensure the proper labeling and purity of the cosmetics marketed in the US. The definition of cosmetics in the US is somewhat narrower than that in the EU. In the US, a cosmetic is defined as a product (excluding pure soap) intended to be applied to the human body for cleansing, beautifying, promoting attractiveness, or altering an appearance. Cosmetics that are imported into the US must comply with the same FDA laws and regulations as those for the cosmetics produced domestically in the US. The FDA conducts label examinations and reviews cosmetic labeling to ensure it is labeled according to FDA laws and regulations. It also reviews the labeling and packaging to ensure it is informative and truthful, with the labeling information provided in English (or Spanish in Puerto Rico) [4].

Certain products regarded as cosmetics in the EU have been classified as over-the-counter (OTC) drugs in the US, including sunscreen products, anti-cavity toothpastes, anti-perspirants, anti-dandruff preparations, skin protectants, and hair restorers. OTC drugs are regulated under the OTC Monograph system for each claimed indication.

The US Federal Food, Drug, and Cosmetic Act does not require cosmetic products and their ingredients to be approved by the FDA before they go on the market, except for color additives that are not intended for use as coal tar hair dyes. However, they must be safe for consumers under the labeled or customary conditions of use. Companies and individuals who market cosmetics have a legal responsibility for the safety of their products and ingredients.

The active ingredients in the respective monographs are evaluated by the agency for safety and efficacy. Those deemed to be safe and effective can be used in products within specified concentration ranges. Sunscreen products and anti-perspirants require additional clinical testing to demonstrate efficacy. Cosmetic colorants, but not hair dyes, are also regulated under US law and require FDA approval, including certified colors and permitted colors. Hair dyes are exempt under the regulations, provided that certain warnings and pre-use testing conditions (testing for sensitization) are mentioned in the product labeling. The safety of all the other cosmetics and their ingredients is the responsibility of the manufacturer.

If a cosmetic has not been evaluated for safety by the manufacturer, it must bear a warning label indicating that the safety has not been substantiated. The FDA has not prescribed how the safety of a product must be substantiated.

The Voluntary Cosmetic Registration Program (VCRP) of the FDA is a reporting system used by manufacturers, packers, and distributors of cosmetic products that are involved in commercial distribution in the US. The VCRP assists the FDA in the regulation of cosmetics by providing information about cosmetic products and their ingredients, their frequency of use, and the firms involved in their manufacture and distribution.

The FDA also collects consumer complaint data from the public and from physicians. This information can be relayed to the manufacturer and/or used to initiate investigations.

In the US, personal care products (PCP) are also regulated under the US Food, Drug and Cosmetic Act, with the FDA responsible for the safety of PCP. Overall, the safety of PCP and their ingredients is the responsibility of the manufacturer. In 1976, the Cosmetic, Toiletry and Fragrance Association (CTFA, presently named the "Personal Care Products Council" or PCPC) established the Cosmetic Ingredient Review (CIR), which provides a mechanism for the self-regulation of the industry.

The CIR provides an independent expert panel to review relevant data on cosmetic ingredients and to decide whether they are safe under their current conditions of use. Voting members of the panel include toxicologists, dermatologists, and chemists from academic institutions, while non-voting members include representatives from the FDA, Consumer Groups, and the PCP industry [5].

The CIR has reviewed the safety of a number of botanical ingredients.

Japanese cosmetics are regulated under the Pharmaceutical and Medical Devices Law (PMDL, formerly the Pharmaceutical Affairs Law), which is supported by a series of subsidiary rules, standards and guidance documents issued by the competent authority, the Ministry of Health, Labor and Welfare (MHLW). The Japanese PMDL requires that a cosmetic should have only mild effects on the human body.

Japan legally classifies cosmetics (in the broad sense, beauty products) into two categories: cosmetics and quasi-drugs. The regulations governing each category differ greatly. Quasi-drugs category includes hair dyes, skin bleaching agents, and hair growth and anti-hair loss agents, is subject to a registration process that requires evidence of efficacy and safety. The details of the registration requirements, which resemble those required for drugs, can be found on the website of the Ministry of Health, Labor and Welfare. In addition, only approved cosmetic ingredients, i.e., those included in an official positive list (CLS = comprehensive licensing standards of cosmetics by category) and corresponding to official specifications, can be used in cosmetics. In recent years, other Asian countries, such as China, South Korea, and Taiwan, have introduced cosmetic regulations similar to those of the Japanese model [6]. In 2010, a safety assessment was officially introduced for cosmetics in China when the former State Food and Drug Administration (SFDA) introduced safety assessment procedures in the management of risky substances that may exist in cosmetics [7].

Although international regulatory schemes on PCP/cosmetics share the same objective, i.e., consumer safety, there are major differences in their approach, particularly in the classification of certain products such as quasi-drugs in Japan or OTC drugs in the US, most of which are classified as cosmetics in the EU. In addition, the recommended safety assessment (oral or dermal toxicity studies, use of alternatives or in vitro tests) is not always consistent [8].

8.1.2 Ban on Animal Testing

The EU implemented a partial ban on the use of animals for the safety evaluation of cosmetic ingredients in 2009, introducing a total ban from 2013 [9].

Countries such as Norway, Iceland, Switzerland, and Liechtenstein followed the EU in implementing this ban.

Many countries have adopted similar bans, such as India, Turkey, Taiwan, South Korea, New Zealand, Guatemala, and, this year, Colombia. In a similar way, the state of California in the USA and in Sao Paulo, Rio de Janeiro and four other states in Brazil. The restriction determines the type of test that should be performed with cosmetics regardless of their natural or synthetic origin.

Although there are many challenges, Chinese authorities have made strides in improving and implementing safety assessments and alternative tests for cosmetics [7].

In 2018, the European Parliament urged for a worldwide ban on the testing of cosmetics on animals by 2023. There are around 40 countries worldwide that have banned or restricted the use of animals for testing cosmetic ingredients. However, there are still a large number of countries where animal testing of cosmetics is still a practice [10].

8.2 SAFETY ASSESSMENT

The use of natural products, more specifically natural cosmetic products, has been increasing. One of the reasons for this is the negative impact of chemicals on the environment and the perception among consumers that natural products have healthier effects [11]. However, natural cosmetics can induce adverse effects, such as sensitization, which is one of the most significant problems observed by dermatologists. Ingredients used in phytocosmetics include plant extracts, expressed juices, tinctures, waxes, vegetable oils, lipids, and essential oils that have different biological activities and are obtained from cultivated or wild plants [12].

Most natural substances are complex mixtures of compounds belonging to various chemical classes, such as alkaloids, lipids, peptides, polyphenols, sugars, and terpenes, among others. The composition of these mixtures can vary depending on the conditions of the plant growth, such as the climate, soil, harvest time or the production methods used. The parts of the plants used usually present different compositions [13].

The number of safety evaluations performed for natural cosmetic ingredients is lower than that for synthetic ingredients.

UNITIS is a professional European organization that unites companies associated with cosmetic ingredients. Due to the lack of information on the safety of botanical ingredients, UNITIS and the Botanical Alliance are currently developing the NCS Tox Project, which involves the creation of a predictive database that determine the toxicological profiles of natural complex substances from plants. The NCS TOX database shall be a major driving force for innovation by tearing down the barriers raised after the complete ban on animal testing and the lack of adequate validated alternative methods to demonstrate the safety of botanical ingredients [14].

The safety assessment of cosmetic ingredients is based on the determination of the margin of safety (MoS), which is the ratio between a Point of Departure (POD) (usually historical no-observed-adverse-effect-level (NOAEL) or benchmark dose (BMD) values from oral toxicity studies) and an estimate of the exposure level. Usually, the NOAEL or the BMD is based on repeated dose toxicity studies in animals and is compared to the dermal exposure level of the ingredient. The NOAEL is defined as the highest dose with no adverse effect in animals. The BMD is the dose that causes a predefined response that is determined by interpolating the data obtained in a dose-response model [15].

The calculated MoS is the assessment factor used in risk and safety assessments to extrapolate information from a group of test animals to humans. A default value of 100 is based on inter- and intra-species differences and a MoS of at least 100 indicates that a cosmetic ingredient is safe for use.

Moreover, when calculating the MoS, it is necessary to have information about the other risks associated with the use of cosmetics such as skin and eye irritations, skin sensitization, dermal absorption, genotoxicity, phototoxicity, carcinogenicity, and reproductive toxicity [16].

Traditionally, all these studies to evaluate the safety of a cosmetic ingredient have involved animals. Therefore, the ban on animal testing has made it necessary to develop alternative methods to evaluate the safety of cosmetics [17].

8.2.1 Alternative Methods and Validation

Different methods have been developed in recent years to evaluate toxicity and safety as alternatives to the traditional animal testing methods, such as *in chemico*, *in vitro*, and *in silico* methods. However, all these methods should be validated before including them for regulatory purposes. Validation ensures that only the test methods that can produce the data that address legislative requirements are accepted as official testing tools and are recognized internationally. This is the case for the methods included in the test guidelines of the Organisation for Economic Co-operation and Development (OECD) [18].

The validation process has been defined by the OECD as:

Test method validation is a process based on scientifically sound principles ... by which the reliability and relevance of a particular test, approach, method, or process are established for a specific purpose. Reliability is defined as the extent of reproducibility of results from a test within and among laboratories over time, when performed using the same standardised protocol. The relevance of a test method describes the relationship between the test and the effect in the target species and whether the test method is meaningful and useful for a defined purpose, with the limitations identified. In brief, it is the extent to which the test method correctly measures or predicts the (biological) effect of interest, as appropriate. Regulatory need, usefulness, and limitations of the test method are aspects of its relevance. New and updated test methods need to be both reliable and relevant, i.e., validated. [19].

The validation of alternative methods is currently conducted in Europe by the European Union Reference Laboratory for alternatives to animal testing (EURL ECVAM). In the USA, the Interagency Coordinating Committee on the Validation of Alternative Methods (ICCVAM) and its supporting National Toxicology Program Interagency Center for the Evaluation of Alternative Toxicological Methods (NICEATM) were established by the Federal Government to work with test developers and federal agencies to facilitate the validation, review, and adoption of new test methods [20]. The other validation centers are in Japan, Korea, Brazil, and Canada [21].

More attention has been paid to the need to replace animal studies in the evaluation of cosmetics due to the ban on animal testing in Europe and other countries.

Different *in vitro* methods had been developed to evaluate the different toxicological effects that should be considered when assessing a synthetic or botanical cosmetic ingredient (Table 8.1). Most of the methods are validated and have been accepted by the regulators. The accepted methods are provided as guidelines on the OECD website and are continually updated with new scientific considerations. The OECD Guidelines for the Testing of Chemicals is a collection of about 150 of the most relevant internationally agreed test methods used by government, industry, and independent laboratories to identify and characterize the potential hazards of chemicals. There are also recommendations from the SCCS regarding the assessment of dermal absorption when studying cosmetic ingredients [22].

8.2.2 Limitations of Some of the *in vitro* Methods

When evaluating the potential toxicity of botanical ingredients using *in vitro* methods, we need to consider possible interferences with the assays before

TABLE 8.1 Cosmetic safety assessment methods

TOXICOLOGICAL EFFECT	IN VITRO METHOD	REFERENCE
Eye irritation	Het-CAM	[23]
	Reconstruted human Cornea-like Ephithelim /RhCE)	[24]
	Bovine Corneal Opacity and Permeability Test Method	[25]
	In vitro Macromolecular Test	[26]
	Isolated Chicken Eye Test Method	[27]
Skin irritation/corrosion	Reconstructed Human Epidermis Test Method	[28]
	In vitro skin corrosion: reconstructed human epidermis (RHE) test method	[29]
	In vitro Membrane Barrier Test	[30]
Sensitization	ARE-Nrf2 Luciferase Test Method	[31]
	In chemico skin sensitization	[32]
Mutagenicity/ Genotoxicity	Bacterial Reverse Mutation Test (Ames test)	[33]
	In vitro Mammalian Cell Micronucleus Test	[34]
	In vitro Mammalian Cell Gene Mutation Test	[35]
	In vitro Mammalian Chromosomal Aberration Test	[36]
Dermal absorption	Skin Absorption: in vitro Method	[37]
Phototoxicity	In vitro 3T3 NRU Phototoxicity Test	[38]
Carcinogenicity	BALB/c 3T3 cell transformation assay	[39]
Reproductive toxicity	Rat whole embryo culture assay	[40]
	Embryonic stem cells assay	[41]
	Zebrafish embryo	[42]
	Micromass assay	[43]

Safety assessment of different botanical ingredients in the literature and evaluated by the SCCS or CIR with the conclusion of the evaluation

BOTANICAL INGREDIENT	CONCLUSION	
Equisetum arvense-derived	Not enough data to support the safety	[59]
Camellia sinensis–Derived Ingredients	Leaf-derived ingredients are safe No data to concluded that non-leaf-derived ingredients are safe	[60]

(Continued)

TABLE 8.1   (*Continued*)

TOXICOLOGICAL EFFECT	IN VITRO METHOD	REFERENCE
Avena sativa (oat)-derived ingredients	The different *A. sativa* ingredients evaluated are safe but the available data are insufficient to support a conclusion of safety for oat meristem cell extract.	[61]
14 Citrus-derived peel oils	Safe for use in cosmetic products when finished products, excluding rinse-off products, do not contain more than 0.0015% (15 ppm) 5-methoxypsoralen	[62]
Spirulina, *Palmaria palmata*, *Cichorium intybus*, and *Medicago sativa* extracts	No harmful effects were confirmed in the acceptability tests	[63]
Acetylated vetiver Oil (AVO) (*Vetiveria zizanioides* root extract acetylated)	AVO with 1% alpha-tocopherol as a fragrance ingredient in cosmetic leave-on and rinse-off type products safe at the concentrations proposed by IFRA: leave-on 0.1% and rinse-off 0.2%	[64]
Cocos nucifera (coconut)-derived ingredients	Not enough data to support the safety	[65]
Aloe vera whole leaf extract	Clear evidence of carcinogenic activity in rats, and was classified by the International Agency for Research on Cancer as a possible human carcinogen (Group 2B).	[66]
Moringa oleifera	No significant irritant potential has been reported from a Patch Test. Good candidate species for sun care and skin-aging protection.	[67]
Citrus spp. Essential oils	With the exception of some phototoxicity of expressed oils, they are generally safe to use with negligible toxicity to humans	[68]
244 Plant-derived fatty acid oils	Safe	[69]
Eugenia dysenterica DC.	Non-phototoxic, non-genotoxic, non-skin irritant, non-skin sensization potential	[70]

TABLE 8.1   (*Continued*)

TOXICOLOGICAL EFFECT	IN VITRO METHOD	REFERENCE
Anthemis nobilis (Roman chamomile)	Safe in the present practices of use and concentration in cosmetics, when formulated to be nonsensitizing.	[71]
Achillea millefolium	extract, flower extract, and flower/leaf/stem extract are safe	[72]
Tagetes minuta and *T. patula* extracts and essential oils	The SCCS considers a maximum level of 0.01% *T. minuta* and *T. patula* extracts and essential oils in leave-on products (except sunscreen cosmetic products) as safe, provided that the alpha terthienyl (terthiophene) content of the *Tagetes* extracts and oils does not exceed 0.35%. *Tagetes* extracts and oils should not be used as ingredients of sunscreen products	[73]
Panax spp. root-derived ingredients	Safe	[74]
Green coffee oil	Safe	[75]
Amino acids from different plants	Safe	[76]
Cucumis sativus (cucumber)-derived ingredients	Safe	[77]
Hypericum perforatum derived ingredients	Safe	[78]
Different phytosterols	Safe in the present practices of use and concentration described in this safety assessment in cosmetics	[79]
Black soybean sprouts	Safe	[80]
Zea mays (corn)	Safe	[81]
Calendulla oficinalis-derived	Safe but may be mild ocular irritant	[82]
Calendulla flower and extract	Safe	[53]
Piper methysticum leaf/root/stem extract	The available data are insufficient to support the safety of these ingredients in cosmetics.	[83]

(*Continued*)

TABLE 8.1 (*Continued*)

TOXICOLOGICAL EFFECT	IN VITRO METHOD	REFERENCE
Ricinus Communis (castor) seed oil and derivatives	Safe	[84]
Capsicum annuum and *C. frutences*	Safe as cosmetics in the practices of use and concentration as described in the safety assessment, when formulated not to be irritating.	[85]
Aloe	*Aloe barbadensis* flower extract, *A. barbadensis* leaf, *A. barbadensis* leaf extract, *A. barbadensis* leaf juice, *A. barbadensis* polysaccharides, and *A. barbadensis* leaf water are safe as cosmetic ingredients in the practices of use and concentrations as described in this safety assessment, if anthraquinone levels in the ingredients do not exceed 50 ppm. The available data are insufficient to support the safety of *Aloe andongensis* extract, *A. andongensis* leaf juice, *Aloe arborescens* leaf extract, *A. arborescens* leaf juice, *Aloe ferox* leaf extract, *A. ferox* leaf juice, or *A. ferox* leaf juice extract in cosmetic products.	[86]
Glycyrrhetinic acid and its salts and esters and glycyrrhizic acid and its salts and esters isolated from licorice plants	Safe	[87]
Rice-derived ingredients	Safe	[88]
Dioscorea villosa (wild yam) root extract	Safe	[89]
PEGs soy sterol	Safe	[90]
Arnica montana extract and *A. montana*	Not enough data to support the safety	[91]

making any conclusion. *In vitro* methods determine the cytotoxic effect of the tested substance through the resazurin conversion assay, which is based on the reduction of resazurin by living cells to the highly fluorescent molecule resorufin. This reduction can be influenced by the anti-oxidant effect of the tested compound, leading to false positive or negative results. Different crude extracts, irrespective of the solvent type, have been shown to diminish the activity of the resazurin assay, resulting in an underestimation of cytotoxicity. Therefore, the resazurin assay is not suitable for the assessment of herbal substance-induced cytotoxicity [44].

The bacterial mutation assay (Ames test) is the first choice for routine genotoxicity screening of chemicals. However, it has long been recognized that materials containing or capable of releasing amino acids can interfere with this assay [45]. Proteins, peptides, and histidine can cause the additional growth of Salmonella bacteria on minimal-medium plates, resulting in additional spontaneous mutations that give rise to false positive results. For this reason, the assay has been modified [40], which is now recommended for the evaluation of botanical substances containing proteins or peptides. Therefore, it is important to know the composition of the plant substances used in cosmetics, as has been pointed out before.

Many plants are known to have ingredients that can cause high sensitization, such as the oil from *Achillea millefolium* [13]. As the formulations made with botanical ingredients are intended for external topical use, allergic contact dermatitis is one of the most prevalent adverse effects associated with their use [46]. The study of the potential sensitization induced by these ingredients is difficult as they are complex mixtures that can interfere with the variety of *in vitro* assays [47]. The methods that study sensitization include the accepted Direct Peptide Reactivity Assay (DPRA) and the Amino acid Derivative Reactivity Assay (ADRA). Both are based on *in chemico* covalent binding to proteins. The correlation between protein reactivity and potential skin sensitization is well established. Since protein reactivity represents only one key event in skin sensitization, the information generated with the test methods developed to address this specific key event may not be sufficient as stand-alone data to make a conclusion about the skin sensitizing potential of chemicals. Moreover, this method does not show enough robustness to assay complex mixtures, especially botanical mixtures, because the test chemicals should be mixed at a specified molecular weight ratio with the synthetic peptides. For this reason, a modification of the *in chemico* screening method using dansyl cysteamine (HTS-DCYA) has been explored for botanical extracts. The data obtained from four plant extracts and known sensitizers suggested that the method can be used to study complex botanical mixtures [48].

A recent study *on in vitro* methods for the evaluation of the sensitizing potential of botanical ingredients was published, using the h-CLAT and KeratinoSens™ methods [49]. The h-CLAT assay is based on the activation of dendritic cells, which express the CD86 and CD54 cell surface proteins following exposure to sensitizers. In the assay THP-1 cells are used as the dendritic cell surrogate and the changes in the expression of CD86 and CD54 induced by the chemicals are measured by flow cytometry. KeratinoSens™ is a cell-based assay measuring luciferase gene induction as an indicator of the activation of the ARE pathway in HaCaT keratinocytes. The results of the study demonstrated the applicability of the two methods in identifying the skin sensitizers present in botanical extracts. The methods show limitations only for oil-based extracts [49].

8.2.3 The Threshold of Toxicological Concern (TTC)

The Threshold of Toxicological Concern (TTC) is a theoretical threshold value for human exposure below which no appreciable risk to human health is expected. It started in 1967 when Frawley proposed a Threshold of Regulation for chemicals intended for use in food packaging materials [50]. This has since evolved into a tiered risk assessment tool. The TTC is based on the concept that safe human exposure levels can be identified for individual substances without determining their toxicological profiles by estimating their toxicity based on their structural similarity to known chemicals. Thus, safe levels of human exposure may be estimated for a substance based on available toxicity data from structurally similar chemicals. In other words, existing knowledge from the World of Chemicals may be applied to estimate the acceptable level of human exposure for a substance under evaluation. The TTC concept has been accepted by national and international regulatory agencies for the safety assessment of substances in the human diet and pharmaceutical preparations. It has also been proposed for chemicals with minimal systemic exposure in humans.

Kroes et al. were the first to explicit discuss how the decision tree could be used for topically and intermittently applied cosmetic ingredients with respect to the chemical domain and route-to-route extrapolation (oral-dermal) [51].

It is difficult to determine POD values, such as the NOAEL values for botanical extracts, which are required for proper risk assessment. The TTC has been proposed as a possible alternative approach for safety evaluations when toxicological information is lacking. A TTC for botanical extracts (Botanical-TTC) in cosmetics has been recently proposed in a meta-analysis based on the PODs derived from the repeated dose toxicity studies of botanical extracts. In the meta-analysis, the POD values for the botanical extracts were obtained from repeated dose toxicity studies in animals that followed OECD test guidelines and the criteria for good laboratory practice. A novel TTC value of 663 µg/day was proposed for botanical extracts [52].

The TTC can be used to evaluate the safety of a complex organic mixture such as a plant part or extract used as a cosmetic ingredient, as is the case for *Callendula*, which has been demonstrated to be safe. However, the composition of the botanical extracts under investigation must be sufficiently documented to apply the TTC concept [53].

8.2.4 Weight of Evidence

There are many publications describing the safety assessment approaches for botanicals based on the history of safe use. However, they do not define what constitutes a history of safe use, which is ultimately subjective. For this reason, a multi-criteria decision analysis (MCDA) has been developed to assess the safety of botanical ingredients using a history of safe use. The model evaluates the similarity of the botanical ingredient of interest to its historic counterpart the comparator, as well as the evidence supporting its history of safe use and any evidence of concern. The assessment made is whether a botanical ingredient is as safe as its comparator that has a history of safe use. To establish compositional similarity between the botanical ingredient and its comparator, an analytical "similarity scoring" approach has been developed [54].

A recent paper highlighted the use of next generation risk assessment, which is defined as an exposure-led, hypothesis-driven risk assessment approach that integrates new approach methodologies (NAMs) to assure safety without the use of animal testing. In the paper, the method was used in a hypothetical safety assessment of 0.1% coumarin in face cream and body lotion (Figure 8.1B). The initial steps involved collating existing data, generating *in silico* predictions, and formulating problems. In parallel, applied and systemic consumer exposure estimates were calculated based on the information on scenarios of use, habits and practices, as well as chemical parameters. A battery of *in vitro* assays was then conducted to characterize the cell response to coumarin. From these data, the POD values and their associated uncertainties were determined. However, the lack of a metabolic capacity of the cell lines used and the potential toxicity of the reactive metabolites led to the generation of additional data. All the POD values were compared with the exposure estimates (plasma Cmax) to calculate the MoS, which was used for the risk assessment [55].

8.2.5 Human Data

For some plant-derived ingredients or products, results from epidemiological and clinical human studies are available on their efficacy and safety and should be taken into account in their risk assessment. All available data, including those on the history of traditional use, should be utilized in the safety assessment of plant-derived ingredients [12].

Controlled clinical studies performed with volunteers include patch tests, open tests, UV protection, among others. Patch tests are useful in determining the type of reaction to a particular cosmetic, whether irritant or allergic. Furthermore, standard test series can help in identifying the agents causing an allergy. In the repeated open application test/provocative use test, the cosmetic test substance is applied twice daily for up to two weeks to an area that is approximately 5 cm^2 on the flexor surface of the forearm near the antecubital area. If no rash appears after one week, the product is considered safe for that individual. This test is applied to screen for allergies to cosmetics, such as fragrances, and to confirm the clinical significance of weak positive patch test reactions. To determine the irritant potential, a panel of 12–20 individuals is used. Patches (material) are applied to the skin (of the back usually) with an occlusive dressing and left undisturbed for a 48-hour period. At the end of the 48-hour period, the patch is removed and the occurrence of any reaction is recorded. The substance being tested is then reapplied to the same site with an occlusive dressing for another 48-hour period. This process is repeated three times a week for either a two- or three-week period. Readings are taken after the removal of each patch. This gives an indication of the potential for cumulated irritation and will reveal very low orders of toxicity.

Finished cosmetic products are usually tested in small populations to confirm their compatibility with skin and mucous membranes and to assess their cosmetic acceptability. Two types of tests are applied in human volunteers: (1) a compatibility test to confirm that there are no harmful effects on the human skin or mucous membrane when a cosmetic product is applied for the first time, and (2) an acceptability test to confirm that expectations are met for a cosmetic product that is in use [56].

Despite the popular belief that natural ingredients are harmless, several cases of adverse reactions to plant extracts have been reported, particularly cutaneous side effects such as allergic contact dermatitis, irritant contact dermatitis, phototoxic reactions, and contact urticaria [57]. However, the number of reported cases of contact dermatitis seems small when compared with the widespread use of botanical remedies. Moreover, little is known about the real incidences of adverse reactions to the botanical extracts present in cosmetics. Therefore, a questionnaire was used in 2,661 volunteers to assess the occurrence of adverse skin reactions with topical botanical preparations, which revealed that contact dermatitis to botanical compounds was possible in ~15% of the declared adverse skin reactions to natural topical products. The most common botanical allergens are propolis, *Compositae* extracts, and *Melaleuca alternifolia* (tea tree) oil [58].

8.3 THE SCCS RECOMMENDATIONS CONCERNING BOTANICAL INGREDIENTS

The SCCS considers the special case of botanicals in the "Notes of Guidance for the Testing of Cosmetic Ingredients and their Safety Evaluation." Considering the changes in composition based on the conditions of plant growth, it is important to know some relevant information such as the qualitative identification, semi-quantitative concentrations, and the International Nomenclature Cosmetic Ingredient (INCI) name if available. The range and maximum levels of the components of mixtures should also be known, while the uses of the ingredient and the recommended maximum concentration should be recorded.

The common or usual names of the plant, variety, species, genus, and family should be indicated and it should be specified if more than one variety of a species is used. Moreover, an organoleptic, macroscopic and microscopic evaluation should be performed to provide a morphological and anatomical description of the plant as well as a photograph, together with a description of the preparation process from collection to preservation.

One of the principal concerns associated with cosmetics is allergic reactions in sensitive consumers. For this reason, there is a list of 26 potentially sensitizing fragrance substances. The presence of these substances must be indicated on the labels of cosmetic products when their concentrations in the final product exceed 0.001% and 0.01% in the leave-on and rinse-off products, respectively [3].

Table 8.1 shows the conclusion from the evaluation of different botanical ingredients.

8.4 CONCLUSIONS

The idea that natural cosmetic ingredients are safer than synthetic ones is not true, as has been observed through the occurrence of adverse effects such as allergies. Therefore, the safety of the botanical cosmetic ingredients should be demonstrated before they can be used, as is the case with other ingredients. The same information file should be prepared for botanical ingredients, with a special emphasis on characterizing the associated plant.

The complexity of botanical ingredients, particularly mixtures of botanical extracts, requires the need for specific methodologies or adaptations of traditional methodologies. The TTC has been proposed as one possible alternative approach for safety evaluation when toxicological information is lacking. The TTC for botanical extracts in cosmetics has been recently proposed.

REFERENCES

1. Ernst, E. Adverse effects of herbal drugs in dermatology. Br J Dermatol. 2000;143(5):923–929.
2. https://eur-lex.europa.eu/legal-content/EN/ALL/?uri=CELEX%3A31976L0768 [accessed 07 December 2020].
3. SCCS (Scientific Committee on Consumer Safety), SCCS Notes of Guidance for the Testing of Cosmetic Ingredients and their Safety Evaluation 10th revision, 24–25 October 2018, SCCS/1602/18. https://ec.europa.eu/health/sites/health/files/scientific_committees/consumer_safety/docs/sccs_o_224.pdf. [accessed 18 November 2020].
4. US FDA (2007). US Food and Drug Administration. Center for Food Safety and Applied Nutrition. Cosmetics. FDA Policy and Authority. Available at: https://www.fda.gov/cosmetics [accessed 17 November 2020].
5. https://www.cir-safety.org [accessed 07 December 2020].
6. Inomata S. Safety assurance of cosmetics in Japan: current situation and future prospects. J Oleo Sci. 2014;63(1):1–6.
7. Luo FY, Su Z, Wu J, et al. The current status of alternative methods for cosmetics safety assessment in China. ALTEX. 2019;36(1):136–9.
8. Nohynek GJ, Antignac E, Re T, et al. Safety assessment of personal care products/cosmetics and their ingredients. Toxicol Appl Pharmacol. 2010;243(2):239–59.
9. Vinardell MP. The use of non-animal alternatives in the safety evaluations of cosmetics ingredients by the Scientific Committee on Consumer Safety (SCCS). Regul Toxicol Pharmacol. 2015;71(2):198–204.
10. New EU Parlamient. 2018. Available at: https://www.europarl.europa.eu/news/en/press-room/20180426IPR02613/testing-cosmetics-on-animals-meps-call-for-worldwide-ban [accessed 17 November 2020].
11. Amberg N, Fogarassy C. Green consumer behavior in the cosmetics market. Resources. 2019; 8.
12. Antignac E, Nohynek GJ, Re T, et al. Safety of botanical ingredients in personal care products/cosmetics. Food Chem Toxicol. 2011;49(2):324–341.
13. Klaschka, U. Naturally toxic: natural substances used in personal care products. Environ Sci Eur. 2015; 27:1–12.

14. http://www.unitis.org [accessed 07 December 2020].
15. EFSA 2009 (European Food Safety Authority). Use of the benchmark dose approach in risk assessment. Guidance of the Scientific Committee. EFSA J. 2009;1150, 1–72.
16. Quantin P, Thélu A, Catoire S, et al. Perspectives and strategies of alternative methods used in the risk assessment of personal care products. Ann Pharm Fr. 2015;73(6):422–35.
17. Adler S, Basketter D, Creton S, et al. Alternative (non-animal) methods for cosmetics testing: current status and future prospects-2010. Arch Toxicol. 2011;85(5):367–485.
18. Griesinger C, Desprez B, Coecke S, et al. Validation of alternative in vitro methods to animal testing: concepts, challenges, processes and tools. Adv Exp Med Biol. 2016;856:65–132.
19. OECD Guidance document on the validation and international acceptance of new or updated test methods for hazard assessment. OECD Series on Testing and Assessment No. 34. ENV/JM/MONO (2005)14. 2005. https://ntp.niehs.nih.gov/iccvam/suppdocs/feddocs/oecd/oecd-gd34.pdf [accessed 23 November 2020].
20. Casey W, Jacobs A, Maull E, et al. A new path forward: the Interagency Coordinating Committee on the Validation of Alternative Methods (ICCVAM) and National Toxicology Program's Interagency Center for the Evaluation of Alternative Toxicological Methods (NICEATM). J Am Assoc Lab Anim Sci. 2015;54(2):170–3.
21. Barroso J, Ahn IY, Caldeira C, et al. International harmonization and cooperation in the validation of alternative methods. Adv Exp Med Biol. 2016;856:343–86.
22. SCCS (Scientific Committee on Consumer Safety), basic criteria for the in vitro assessment of dermal absorption of cosmetic ingredients, 22 June 2010. Available at: https://ec.europa.eu/health/scientific_committees/consumer_safety/docs/sccs_s_002.pdf. [accessed 18 November 2020].
23. Steiling W, Bracher M, Courtellemont P, et al. The HET-CAM, a useful in vitro assay for assessing the eye irritation properties of cosmetic formulations and ingredients. Toxicol In Vitro. 1999. 13(2):375–84.
24. OECD 2019, Test No. 492: Reconstructed human Cornea-like Epithelium (RhCE) test method for identifying chemicals not requiring classification and labelling for eye irritation or serious eye damage, OECD Guidelines for the Testing of Chemicals, Section 4, OECD Publishing, Paris, https://doi.org/10.1787/9789264242548-en. [accessed 23 November 2020].
25. OECD 2020, Test No. 437: Bovine Corneal Opacity and Permeability Test Method for Identifying i) Chemicals Inducing Serious Eye Damage and ii) Chemicals Not Requiring Classification for Eye Irritation or Serious Eye Damage, OECD Guidelines for the Testing of Chemicals, Section 4, OECD Publishing, Paris, https://doi.org/10.1787/9789264203846-en. [accessed 23 November 2020].
26. OECD 2019, Test No. 496: In vitro Macromolecular Test Method for Identifying Chemicals Inducing Serious Eye Damage and Chemicals Not Requiring Classification for Eye Irritation or Serious Eye Damage, OECD Guidelines for the Testing of Chemicals, Section 4, OECD Publishing, Paris, https://doi.org/10.1787/970e5cd9-en. [accessed 23 November 2020].

27. OECD 2018, Test No. 438: Isolated Chicken Eye Test Method for Identifying i) Chemicals Inducing Serious Eye Damage and ii) Chemicals Not Requiring Classification for Eye Irritation or Serious Eye Damage, OECD Guidelines for the Testing of Chemicals, Section 4, OECD Publishing, Paris, https://doi.org/10.1787/9789264203860-en. [accessed 23 November 2020].

28. OECD 2020, Test No. 439: *In Vitro* Skin Irritation: Reconstructed Human Epidermis Test Method, OECD Guidelines for the Testing of Chemicals, Section 4, OECD Publishing, Paris, https://doi.org/10.1787/9789264242845-en. [accessed 23 November 2020].

29. OECD 2019, Test No. 431: *In vitro* skin corrosion: reconstructed human epidermis (RHE) test method, OECD Guidelines for the Testing of Chemicals, Section 4, OECD Publishing, Paris, https://doi.org/10.1787/9789264264618-en. [accessed 23 November 2020].

30. OECD 2015, Test No. 435: *In Vitro* Membrane Barrier Test Method for Skin Corrosion, OECD Guidelines for the Testing of Chemicals, Section 4, OECD Publishing, Paris https://doi.org/10.1787/9789264242791-en. [accessed 23 November 2020].

31. OECD 2018, Test No. 442D: *In Vitro* Skin Sensitisation: ARE-Nrf2 Luciferase Test Method, OECD Guidelines for the Testing of Chemicals, Section 4, OECD Publishing, Paris, https://doi.org/10.1787/9789264229822-en [accessed 23 November 2020].

32. OECD 2020, Test No. 471: Bacterial Reverse Mutation Test, OECD Guidelines for the Testing of Chemicals, Section 4, OECD Publishing, Paris, https://doi.org/10.1787/9789264071247-en. [accessed 23 November 2020].

33. OECD 2020, Test No. 442C: *In Chemico* Skin Sensitisation: Assays addressing the Adverse Outcome Pathway key event on covalent binding to proteins, OECD Guidelines for the Testing of Chemicals, Section 4, OECD Publishing, Paris, https://doi.org/10.1787/9789264229709-en. [accessed 23 November 2020].

34. OECD 2016, Test No. 490: *In Vitro* Mammalian Cell Gene Mutation Tests Using the Thymidine Kinase Gene, OECD Guidelines for the Testing of Chemicals, Section 4, OECD Publishing, Paris, https://doi.org/10.1787/9789264264908-en. [accessed 23 November 2020].

35. OECD 2016, Test No. 487: *In Vitro* Mammalian Cell Micronucleus Test, OECD Guidelines for the Testing of Chemicals, Section 4, OECD Publishing, Paris, https://doi.org/10.1787/9789264264861-en. [accessed 23 November 2020].

36. OECD 2016, Test No. 473: *In Vitro* Mammalian Chromosomal Aberration Test, OECD Guidelines for the Testing of Chemicals, Section 4, OECD Publishing, Paris, https://doi.org/10.1787/9789264264649-en. [accessed 23 November 2020].

37. OECD 2004, Test No. 428: Skin Absorption: *In Vitro* Method, OECD Guidelines for the Testing of Chemicals, Section 4, OECD Publishing, Paris, https://doi.org/10.1787/9789264071087-en. https://www.oecd-ilibrary.org/environment/test-no-428-skin-absorption-in-vitro-method_9789264071087-en. [accessed 23 November 2020].

38. OECD 2019, Test No. 432: *In Vitro* 3T3 NRU Phototoxicity Test, OECD Guidelines for the Testing of Chemicals, Section 4, OECD Publishing, Paris, https://doi.org/10.1787/9789264071162-en. [accessed 23 November 2020].

39. Sasaki K, Bohnenberger S, Hayashi K, et al. Recommended protocol for the BALB/c 3T3 cell transformation assay. Mutat Res. 2012;744(1):30–5.

40. Thompson C, Morley P, Kirkland D, et al. Modified bacterial mutation test procedures for evaluation of peptides and amino acid-containing material. Mutagenesis. 2005;20(5):345–50.
41. Panzica-Kelly JM, Brannen KC, Ma Y, et al. Establishment of a molecular embryonic stem cell developmental toxicity assay. Toxicol Sci. 2013; 131(2):447–57.
42. Brannen K.C., Charlap J.H., Lewis E.M. Zebrafish Teratogenicity Testing. In: Barrow P. (eds) Teratogenicity Testing. Methods in Molecular Biology (Methods and Protocols), vol 947. Humana Press, Totowa, NJ.; 2013:383–401.
43. Spézia F, Barrow PC. The teratology testing of cosmetics. Methods Mol Biol. 2013;947:91–4.
44. Cordier W, and Steenkamp V. Evaluation of Four Assays to Determine Cytotoxicity of Selected Crude Medicinal Plant Extracts In vitro. J Pharm Res Int. 2015; 7(1):16–21.
45. Busch DB, Bryan GT. Presence and measurement of sample histidine in the Ames test: quantification and possible elimination of a source of false-positive mutagenicity test results. Environ Mol Mutagen. 1987;10(4):397–410.
46. Uter W, Schmidt E, Geier J, et al. Contact allergy to essential oils: current patch test results (2000–2008) from the Information Network of Departments of Dermatology (IVDK). Contact Dermatitis. 2010; 63:277–83.
47. Baell, J. B. Feeling nature's PAINS: natural products, natural product drugs, and pan assay interference compounds (PAINS). J Nat Prod. 2016; 79: 616–28.
48. Avonto C, Chittiboyina AG, Sadrieh N, et al. In chemico skin sensitization risk assessment of botanical ingredients. J Appl Toxicol. 2018;38(7):1047–53.
49. Nishijo T, Miyazawa M, Saito K, et al. Sensitivity of KeratinoSens™ and h-CLAT for detecting minute amounts of sensitizers to evaluate botanical extract. J Toxicol Sci. 2019;44(1):13–21.
50. Frawley JP. Scientific evidence and common sense as a basis for food-packaging regulations. Food Cosmet Toxicol 1967;5(3):293–308.
51. Kroes R, Renwick AG, Feron V, et al. Application of the threshold of toxicological concern (TTC) to the safety evaluation of cosmetic ingredients. Food Chem Toxicol. 2007;45(12):2533–62
52. Kawamoto T, Fuchs A, Fautz R, et al. Threshold of toxicological concern (TTC) for botanical extracts (botanical-TTC) derived from a meta-analysis of repeated-dose toxicity studies. Toxicol Lett. 2019;316:1–9.
53. Re TA, Mooney D, Antignac E, et al. Application of the threshold of toxicological concern approach for the safety evaluation of calendula flower (Calendula officinalis) petals and extracts used in cosmetic and personal care products. Food Chem Toxicol. 2009;47(6):1246–54
54. Neely T, Walsh-Mason B, Russell P, et al. A multi-criteria decision analysis model to assess the safety of botanicals utilizing data on history of use. Toxicol Int. 2011;18(1):S20–9.
55. Baltazar MT, Cable S, Carmichael PL, et al. A next-generation risk assessment case study for coumarin in cosmetic products. Toxicol Sci. 2020;176(1):236–252.
56. Nigam PK. Adverse reactions to cosmetics and methods of testing. Indian J Dermatol Venereol Leprol. 2009 75(1):10–8.
57. Kiken D A, Cohen D E. Contact dermatitis to botanical extracts. Am J Contact Dermat. 2002;13:148–52.

58. Corazza M, Borghi A, Gallo R, et al. Topical botanically derived products: use, skin reactions, and usefulness of patch tests. A multicentre Italian study. Contact Dermat. 2014;70(2):90–7.

59. CIR Safety Assessment of *Equisetum arvense*-derived Ingredients as Used in Cosmetics 2020. Available at: https://www.cir-safety.org/sites/default/files/equise062020slr.pdf. [accessed 18 November 2020]

60. Becker LC, Bergfeld WF, Belsito DV, et al. Safety assessment of *Camellia sinensis*-derived ingredients as used in cosmetics. Int J Toxicol. 2019;38(3):48S–70S.

61. Becker LC, Bergfeld WF, Belsito DV, et al. Safety assessment of *Avena sativa* (Oat)-derived ingredients as used in cosmetics. Int J Toxicol. 2019;38(3):23S–47S.

62. Burnett CL, Fiume MM, Bergfeld WF, et al. Safety assessment of citrus-derived peel oils as used in cosmetics. Int J Toxicol. 2019; 38(2): 33S–59S.

63. Campos PMBGM, Benevenuto CG, Calixto LS, et al. *Spirulina, Palmaria Palmata, Cichorium Intybus,* and *Medicago sativa* extracts in cosmetic formulations: an integrated approach of *in vitro* toxicity and *in vivo* acceptability studies. Cutan Ocul Toxicol. 2019;38(4):322–29.

64. SCCS members; External experts. Opinion of the Scientific Committee on consumer safety (SCCS) – final opinion on the safety of fragrance ingredient Acetylated Vetiver Oil (AVO) - (*Vetiveria zizanioides* root extract acetylated) - Submission III. Regul Toxicol Pharmacol. 2019;107:104389.

65. CIR Safety Assessment of *Cocos nucifera* (Coconut)-Derived Ingredients as Used in Cosmetics. 2019. Available at: https://www.cir-safety.org/supplementaldoc/safety-assessment-cocos-nucifera-coconut-derived-ingredients-used-cosmetics. [accessed 18 November 2020].

66. Guo X, Mei N. *Aloe vera*: a review of toxicity and adverse clinical effects. J Environ Sci Health C Environ Carcinog Ecotoxicol Rev. 2016;34(2): 77–96.

67. Baldisserotto A, Buso P, Radice M, et al. *Moringa oleifera* leaf extracts as multifunctional ingredients for "Natural and Organic" sunscreens and photoprotective preparations. Molecules. 2018;23(3):664.

68. Dosoky NS, Setzer WN. Biological activities and safety of *Citrus* spp. essential oils. Int J Mol Sci. 2018;19(7):1966.

69. Burnett CL, Fiume MM, Bergfeld WF, et al. Safety assessment of plant-derived fatty acid oils. Int J Toxicol. 2017; 36(3): 51S–129S.

70. Moreira LC, de Ávila RI, Veloso DFMC, et al. In vitro safety and efficacy evaluations of a complex botanical mixture of *Eugenia dysenterica* DC. (Myrtaceae): prospects for developing a new dermocosmetic product. Toxicol In Vitro. 2017;45(3):397–408.

71. Johnson W Jr, Heldreth B, Bergfeld WF, et al. Safety assessment of *Anthemis nobilis*-derived ingredients as used in cosmetics. Int J Toxicol. 2017;36(1):57S–66S.

72. Becker LC, Bergfeld WF, Belsito DV et al. Safety assessment of *Achillea millefolium* as used in cosmetics. Int J Toxicol. 2016;35(3):5S–15S.

73. SCCS (Scientific Committee on Consumer Safety), Coenraads PJ. Opinion of the Scientific Committee on Consumer Safety (SCCS) – opinion on the fragrance ingredients *Tagetes minuta* and *Tagetes patula* extracts and essential oils (phototoxicity only) in cosmetic products. Regul Toxicol Pharmacol. 2016;76:213–4.

74. Becker LC, Bergfeld WF, Belsito DV, et al. Safety assessment of *Panax* spp root-derived ingredients as used in cosmetics. Int J Toxicol 2015; 34(3) 5S–42S.
75. Wagemaker TA, Rijo P, Rodrigues LM, et al. Integrated approach in the assessment of skin compatibility of cosmetic formulations with green coffee oil. Int J Cosmet Sci. 2015;37(5):506–10.
76. Burnett C, Heldreth B, Bergfeld WB et al. Safety assessment of animal- and plant-derived amino acids as used in cosmetics. Int J Toxicol. 2014; 33(4): 5S–12S.
77. Fiume MM, Bergfeld WF, Belsito DV, et al. Safety assessment of *Cucumis sativus* (Cucumber)-derived ingredients as used in cosmetics. Int J Toxicol. 2014;33(2):47S–64S.
78. Becker LC, Bergfeld WF, Belsito DV, et al. Amended safety assessment of *Hypericum perforatum*-derived ingredients as used in cosmetics. Int J Toxicol. 2014;33(3):5S–23S.
79. CIR Safety Assessment of Phytosterols as Used in Cosmetics. 2013. Available at: https://www.cir-safety.org/supplementaldoc/safety-assessment-phytosterols-used-cosmetics-1. [accessed 18 November 2020].
80. Lai J, Xin C, Zhao Y et al. Study of active ingredients in black soybean sprouts and their safety in cosmetic use. Molecules. 2012; 17:11669–79.
81. Andersen FA, Bergfeld WF, Belsito DV, et al. Final report of the safety assessment of cosmetic ingredients derived from *Zea mays* (corn). Int J Toxicol. 2011;30(3):17S–39S.
82. Andersen FA, Bergfeld WF, Belsito DV, et al. Final report of the cosmetic ingredient review expert panel amended safety assessment of *Calendula officinalis*–derived cosmetic ingredients. Int J Toxicol. 2010;29(6 suppl):221S–243S.
83. Robinson V, Bergfeld WF, Belsito DV, et al. Final report on the safety assessment of *Piper methysticum* leaf/root/stem extract and *Piper methysticum* root extract. Int J Toxicol. 2009;28(6):175S–88S.
84. CIR. Final report on the safety assessment of *Ricinus Communis* (Castor) seed oil, hydrogenated castor oil, glyceryl ricinoleate, glyceryl ricinoleate se, ricinoleic acid, potassium ricinoleate, sodium ricinoleate, zinc ricinoleate, cetyl ricinoleate, ethyl ricinoleate, glycol ricinoleate, isopropyl ricinoleate, methyl ricinoleate, and octyldodecyl ricinoleate. Int J Toxicol. 2007;26(3):31–77.
85. CIR. Final report on the safety assessment of *Capsicum annuum* extract, *Capsicum annuum* fruit extract, *Capsicum annuum* resin, *Capsicum annuum* fruit powder, *Capsicum frutescens* fruit, *Capsicum frutescens* fruit extract, *Capsicum frutescens* resin, and capsaicin. Int J Toxicol. 2007;26(1):3–106.
86. CIR. Final report on the safety assessment of *Aloe andongensis* Extract, Aloe *Aloe andongensis* Leaf Juice, *Aloe arborescens* Leaf Extract, *Aloe arborescens* Leaf Juice, *Aloe arborescens* Leaf Protoplasts, *Aloe barbadensis* Flower Extract, *Aloe barbadensis* Leaf, *Aloe barbadensis* Leaf Extract, *Aloe barbadensis* Leaf Juice, *Aloe barbadensis* Leaf Polysaccharides, *Aloe barbadensis* Leaf Water, *Aloe ferox* Leaf Extract, *Aloe ferox* Leaf Juice, and *Aloe ferox* Leaf Juice Extract. Int J Toxicol. 2007;26(2):1–50.
87. CIR. Final report on the safety assessment of glycyrrhetinic acid, potassium glycyrrhetinate, disodium succinoyl glycyrrhetinate, glyceryl glycyrrhetinate, glycyrrhetinyl stearate, stearyl glycyrrhetinate, glycyrrhizic acid, ammonium glycyrrhizate, dipotassium glycyrrhizate, disodium glycyrrhizate, trisodium glycyrrhizate, methyl glycyrrhizate, and potassium glycyrrhizinate. Int J Toxicol. 2007;26(2):79–112.

88. CIR. Amended final report on the safety assessment of *Oryza sativa* (rice) bran oil, *Oryza sativa* (rice) germ oil, rice bran acid, *Oryza sativa* (rice) bran wax, hydrogenated rice bran wax, *Oryza sativa* (rice) bran extract, *Oryza sativa* (rice) extract, *Oryza sativa* (rice) germ powder, *Oryza sativa* (rice) starch, *Oryza sativa* (rice) bran, hydrolyzed rice bran extract, hydrolyzed rice bran protein, hydrolyzed rice extract, and hydrolyzed rice protein. Int J Toxicol. 2006;25(2):91–120.

89. CIR. Final report of the amended safety assessment of *Dioscorea villosa* (Wild Yam) root extract. Int J Toxicol. 2004;23(2):49–54.

90. CIR. Final report of the amended safety assessment of PEG-5, -10, -16, -25, -30, and -40 soy sterol. Int J Toxicol. 2004;23(2):23–47.

91. CIR. Final report on the safety assessment of *Arnica montana* extract and *Arnica montana*. Int J Toxicol. 2001;20(2):1–11

Sustainable Phytocosmetics

9

Sharna-kay Daley and
Geoffrey A. Cordell

Contents

9.1 INTRODUCTION

In 2015, the United Nations General Assembly introduced the 17 goals for sustainable development (SDGs) for 2030. These are universal goals, wherein every nation and every sector of society is challenged to act. They focus on integration and inter-connectedness (one goal is not isolated from the others); they seek creative transformations in lifestyle and recommend significant changes in the way that humans interact with the Earth [1].

Nearly all 17 SDGs impinge on sustainable phytocosmetics. The most prominent are: sustainable agriculture, promoting health and well-being, education and life-long learning, sustainable economic growth, industrialized innovation, sustainable consumption, combatting climate change, conserving and managing global terrestrial and marine natural resources, and establishing global partnerships. The SDGs are a call for creativity and innovation in all sectors; an opportunity to examine pathways, practices, inputs, and outcomes, and to challenge those activities with improvement. They are a call to enhance the quality of our thinking and acting. Many years ago, Deming made such transformations abundantly clear with "Quality begins with intent" [2]. Newton calls for "Deep Work," a time for creative thinking, individually and collectively, about pathways forward [3]. How does this apply to sustainable phytocosmetics?

Sustainability is a conscious practice for utilizing natural resources that meets current needs without jeopardizing their availability for future generations, and considers the economic and social aspects of the practice [4, 5]. For many years, the cosmetic industry has engaged in programs to enhance the scientific, environmental, and societal obligations of its operations and products. This, in response to a marketplace demanding the "greening" of processes, sustainability in marketed products, and enhanced corporate social responsibility [6, 7]. Regulatory aspects, particularly in the European Union (see Chapter 8), concerning the design and packaging of materials, labeling requirements, and the demands of consumers, are evoking enhanced corporate transparency and accountability [8]. Simply put, there is a "green" revolution underway in the personal care industry.

The 5,000 years of cosmetic use reflect the sustained application of natural products on the skin for various purposes [9–11]. Cosmetic products from ancient times, such as henna (mehndi on the Indian subcontinent) from the leaves of *Lawsonia inermis* L. (Lythraceae), fragrant essential oils, such as lavender oil [*Lavendula angustifolia* Mill. (Lamiaceae)], or the 2,000 year-old production of cochineal for lipsticks and rouge, are testament to the continuous cultivation of plants and rearing of insects for cosmetic use. In the past

40 years, business innovation and market expansion in the cosmetics industry has focused on developing a positive relationship with health care and wellness, including modulating the effects of the ageing process, internally and externally [12–14]. Products for slowing ageing through anti-oxidants [15], based on the biological role of reactive oxygen species (ROS) [16–18], became an enormous innovation opportunity. Together with other biological effects, this led to the term "cosmeceutical," a cosmetic with a healing action, as proposed in 1984 by Kligman [19, 20].

Interest in plant anti-oxidant activity has expanded dramatically [21–23]. It is anticipated that most plants will show anti-oxidant potential due to the ubiquitous presence of catechol (1,2-dihydroxyphenol) units in their flavonoids, isoflavonoids, polyphenolics, tannins, etc. [24–26]. Ascorbic acid, lycopene, and some essential oil monoterpenes are rare non-phenolic anti-oxidants [27–29]. To justify developing anti-oxidants as sustainable, healthy additives for cosmeceuticals, target assays (for ageing, melanoma, and acne) must be utilized using appropriate secondary assays to identify specific plants for sustainable development [30, 31].

In addition to anti-oxidants, cosmeceuticals embrace anti-carcinogens, anti-inflammatory agents, skin whitening agents, photoprotective agents, colorants, essential oils, hair growth promotors, moisturizing agents, surfactants, and thickening agents. They may target a range of skin conditions, including photo-damage [32], hyperpigmentation [33], acne [34, 35], oily skin [36, 37], dandruff [38], or rosacea [39, 40], as well as for hair growth [41, 42]. These functional characterizations coalesce with the patient-desired attributes of appearance, physical and mental health benefits, and a "greener" product composition and presentation [43–50].

Based on the SDGs, "sustainable," and the myriad of creative expressions and innovations associated with it, will be approached in several different ways. "Sustainable" for a plant reflects constituent origin, production, long-term availability, and its packaging in products. It applies to reliability and consistency, implying that quality control is applied from the point of origin to the consumer and beyond, independent of timeframe. Sustainable for the consumer applies to the promotion of well-being; and the on-going physiological and psychological benefits from cosmetic use. Continual product innovation is an economic driver for new and established industries; the core of sustainable development. Other SDG aspects include assuring total ingredient availability that considers energy use and water supplies. Examining the impact of production technologies on climate change, and in the obverse, the impact of climate change on the quality of the plant materials, are important considerations, together with critically evaluating the phyto- and marine constituent sourcing for optimal sustainability. This chapter looks at the challenges concerning the sustainability of phytocosmetics, particularly with respect to regulations in the production phases, accessibility and disposability, considering also the evolving greener expectations of the contemporary consumer.

9.2 COSMETICS AND THEIR "GREEN" ASSESSMENT – SOURCING, PROCESSING, AND PRODUCTION

9.2.1 Sourcing and Processing: Agricultural and Development Aspects

Of the approximately 393,000 vascular plants, about 28,187 have been used for biological purposes [51], and at least 85% of these are wild-crafted. Prior to terrestrial or marine wild-crafting, local regulatory considerations related to the Convention on Biological Diversity and the Nagoya Protocol must be respected, including the conservation and sustainable use of the biodiversity, and the fair and equitable sharing of benefits arising from the acquired genetic resources. Permissions and negotiations for access, which may be different for research and production purposes, are pre-conditions [52]. Authentication of the wild-crafted or cultivated species requires an established system for positive identification through micro- and macroscopy and DNA-based barcoding [53, 54].

Recommendations for plant collection for cosmetics and cosmeceuticals were made in the WHO Guidelines on Good Agricultural and Collection Practices for Medicinal Plants [55], and the promotion of conservation and sustainability have been described [56]. In addition, the International Standard for Sustainable Wild Collection of Medicinal and Aromatic Plants (ISSC-MAP) [57] has six major principles: (i) maintaining wild MAP resources, (ii) preventing negative environmental impact, (iii) abiding by legal and ethical requirements, (iv) respecting customary rights and practices, (v) applying responsible management practices, and (vi) having responsible business practices.

As demand increases, the relationship between the *in situ* or in-field conservation of traded species becomes an important aspect of sustainable development. Consumer desires which favor "natural," holistic sourcing compared with cultivation can lead to the threat of an endangered species [58]. Collection of bark and roots from perennials and trees versus leaves and flowers or fruits has very different implications for sustainable practices, as well as biological outcomes. Continuing to wild-harvest plants poses other significant issues, particularly regarding species range, population status, and optimal harvesting times. Sustainability considerations must involve the synergistic relationship between the people, plants, and the ecology, or the local society itself may not be sustainable. Management of "open access" plant resources to prevent over-harvesting is challenging, and more government-led initiatives to promote conserved wild-harvesting areas which can provide a sustainable resource to the local community for economic development, are required to counter urbanization losses [59, 60]. However, transition to large-scale cultivation may eliminate a thriving community trading tradition, which negatively impacts local economic development [61]. Promotion of the cultivation and responsible use of plants [62] focuses on the balance between conservation (and possible regulatory over-protection) and the responsible scientific exploration of economic value through sustainable development [63]. This conservation through promoting crop implementation was recognized as of community importance in Nepal to enrich local livelihood [64].

Following an assessment [65], a business model study of the commercial plant dynamics in Uttarakhand State in northwest India with all stakeholders (policymakers, growers, collectors, traders, and manufacturers) [66] showed that the existing practices were "opportunistic" and "inconsistent" with conservation and stakeholder economics, and led to valuable stakeholder initiatives in line with several SDGs. These included: (i) motivating and guiding local growers to prioritize mass cultivation of valuable plants with determined bioactivity, (ii) establishing a value chain with financial responsibilities based on volume and commercial interest, locally and internationally, (iii) developing marketing practices which match the cultivation program, (iv) improving the level of agricultural, scientific, and business acumen in the local decision-making processes, and (v) enhancing local and national public awareness of the attributes of the plants. However, the disappearance of valuable plants due to overharvesting from wild resources [67] remains a major global concern [68–73]. Sustainable sourcing based on cultivation, which improved the quality of lavender fields around the world [74–76], attests to the value, biologically and economically, of a highly reproducible starting material.

The "quality" of any phytoconstituent matrix (metabolome) begins in the field, whether the plant is acquired through cultivation or wild-crafting. Sustainable quality from field to store to dresser, probably over an extended time-line, involving producers, collectors, processors, manufacturers, and distributors, must embrace standardized assessment protocols applied at each procedural step to provide a consistent and sustainable product. As blockchain technology (*vide infra*) for traded plants evolves as an industry standard, accurate scientific information relating to the quality of the materials at each transaction will be essential. Integration of information systems, botany, chemistry, and biology can form a sustainable quality control management protocol, with supportive and relevant, reproducible analytical techniques and biological assays [77–79].

Variability in plant metabolite profiles of collected and cultivated plants led to numerous studies of tissue culture, cell-based, and cell-free systems for commercially important compounds and extracts for the cosmetic industry, especially for the more desirable, eco-friendly products [80]. Since efficacy based on a specific dose is less relevant for a topical cosmeceutical, metabolite titer levels are of lower importance, although maintaining a standardized metabolite profile is necessary [81]. Numerous plant cell culture-derived preparations are now incorporated into various cosmetic products [82], including for skin rejuvenation and wound healing [83–85], treatment of rosacea and acne [86, 87], and hair loss [88]. The significant impact of plant cell cultures in the sustainable development of new cosmetic products has been reviewed [84, 89–92].

What is identified in the DNA bar-coding process is typically more than the plant collected for the phytocosmetic. The Latin binomial, usually regulated for the product label, does not represent genomics of the whole plant. Neither does it reflect modulations in the metabolite profile through changing geolocation, such as soil pH, fertility, water, sunlight, temperature, pests, fungal disease, herbivory, and the plant endophytes [93–96]. Any changes in the metabolite profile from an established standard preparation will alter the biological outcomes. This may impact the volume of plant material needed to reach a standardized product positively or negatively. Looking to a sustainable future, research is essential for the impacts of climate change on the metabolite profiles of commercially significant medicinal and essential oil plants. Specifically, changes due to modulations in rainfall, heat, UV radiation, elevated ozone levels, and enhanced salinity from rising sea levels require detailed investigation [97].

9.2.2 Production: Regulations and Sustainability

The United States Food and Drug Administration (USFDA) does not recognize the term "cosmeceutical"; it has no meaning in Federal law. Consequently, the USFDA does not "approve" such items, unless the manufacturer makes therapeutic claims in a drug category [98]. Individual cosmetic and cosmeceutical products may be voluntarily "registered" at the USFDA under the Voluntary Cosmetic Registration Program (VCRP); however, that does not represent approval of the product. There are three main Acts which apply to cosmetics in the United States: the Federal Food, Drug, and Cosmetic Act (FD&CA), the Fair Packaging and Labeling Act (FPLA), and the Dietary Supplement Health and Education Act (DSHEA) of 1994, which regulates manufacture and labeling of dietary supplements, but not the content. None of the three acts address the sustainability or biodegradation issues of what is being regulated. On the other hand, the term "organic," which is often indicated on the labels of phytocosmetics, has specific legal meaning in Federal law under the authority of the US Department of Agriculture (USDA); an item with >95% organic ingredients may be labeled as "organic," with the certifying agent details indicated. However, such a designation bears no relationship to product QSECA, or to sustainability.

The responsibilities for the content of the product, and thus for cosmetic and cosmeceutical quality control and its sustainability remain with the manufacturer, solely on a trust basis. This is antithetical to the preferred notion of sustainable development, harmonized international standards, transparent certification, and product monitoring to protect the consumer/patient from flagrant fraud and/or retail and on-line products which do not meet acceptable standards. A more enlightening level of label (and website) disclosure is necessary [99–102]. The global unknown relating to sustainability, and to the quality control of cosmetics and cosmeceuticals, is the range of on-line products, often promoted with medical and physical claims, for materials of unknown provenance. Illegal claims of prevention, treatment, and cure were evident in the advertising of 55% of on-line of orally consumed dietary supplements [103]; a corresponding survey of on-line cosmeceuticals would be illuminating.

Japan is the only country having specific regulatory oversight for cosmeceuticals [104], and at least 40 countries in Europe, Asia, and South America, have much stricter regulations for cosmetic constituents than the United States [105]. A harmonious alignment of regulations would assist all stakeholders in encouraging innovation, entrepreneurism, more sustainable production methods and material consistency across global markets in line with the SDGs [106]. Business entities, and, more importantly, the consumer/patient, would benefit from resolution of the fundamental differences between the European Union Cosmetics Regulations (discussed in Chapter 8) and the USFDA framework for cosmetics and cosmeceuticals, and foster sustainable economic development [107–109]. A significant global issue is that basic international standards, even regional standards, for cosmetics and cosmeceuticals are minimal or non-existent. Protecting the consumer/patient from unsubstantiated claims and fraud, including those made for on-line products, while maintaining the pursuit of sustainable development goals for phytocosmetic plants for societal health and conservation of resources, should be a major industry concern.

9.2.3 Production: Greening of Products and Sustainability

The cosmeceuticals market is considered the fastest growing (9–10% annually) sector of the personal care industry [110]. Besides product innovation, the dramatic market growth in the past 25 years is related to the strong desire from consumers for "natural" products, an evolving "greening" process in industry, and enhanced, evidence-based research. As a consumer, Quality, Safety, Efficacy, Consistency, and Accessibility (availability and affordability), summarized as **QSECA**, is a target for an ideal product. What those factors represent, how they are achieved sustainably, the regulatory background, and the responsibility to ensure those attributes long-term, have been discussed [99–101, 111].

Increasing societal and corporate concerns regarding "natural" products and the environment are affecting our lives in many ways. "Old" practices are no longer acceptable, and the impact of environmentally unfriendly manufacturing protocols on the condition of the Earth is being critically assessed [112]. The development of sustainable practices regarding solvents and energy usage within "green chemistry" [113, 114] inspires creativity. Transitioning from plastics which take hundreds of years to degrade to those that biodegrade more rapidly is an example [115, 116]. Developing sustainable solutions in the cosmetic industry to multiple challenges represents innovation, in the product contents, including their acquisition and processing, for the packaging, for post-use disposition, corporate business practices, and marketing [117, 118]. Continuing evolution will, if the consumer is the priority, redefine these attributes, and the nature and sustainability of the available products in the marketplace.

The binomial of the plant(s) in the product is not a concern for the consumer; more significant are the biological effects [99]. Like *Capsicum annuum* L. (Solanaceae) and the "hotness" of the chili peppers, the biological response of any plant used for cosmetic or cosmeceutical purposes may vary considerably. Analytical studies, usually UPLC-MS^n-based metabolomics [119–120], are necessary to develop and establish a consistent standard that over time is sustainable, and independent of source. Biological assessment becomes important to establish which chemovariant is preferred for the application, as that may reflect on the volume of plant material to be used, and promotes the establishment of a sustainable, effective, and consistent plant supply protocol.

Because a material is from nature, it is not necessarily safe, a common misconception. Which brings us to some myths, developed related to traditional medicine, whether for treatment *per se*, or incorporated into a cosmetic product [102, 111]. One fundamental myth is that because the plant or essential oil has been used for hundreds (or even thousands) of years that it is both "safe" and "effective." Another myth suggests that the constituents are always the same, irrespective of the origin of the material, the plant part, or the extraction method. Other myths concern the age of the plant (older is less effective), collection (wild-crafted is more active), constituent analysis (complex matrices cannot be standardized), and that the plant (and the associated indigenous knowledge) will always be there.

Historical evidence of the human use of plants is not based on a standardized sample using appropriate controls, and therefore lacks experimental reproducibility. Dealing with these "myths" requires contemporary scientific evidence using material that is supplied in a sustainable, reproducible manner. An extraction process might now be "greener" and display a quite different metabolite and biological profile from the original preparation. In the United States, there is no legal requirement to disclose a complete list of ingredients, their origin, or the processing method on a cosmetic product label or corporate website [121]. Consequently, the health-conscious consumer is effectively blinded to the contents and their relationship to a sustainable origin; interestingly, so also is the government. This "regulatory obsolescence" [122] is especially unacceptable for cosmeceuticals, for which health beneficent effects are a marketing hallmark.

Sustainability is also a factor in biological assessment. Namely, the testing methods (*in vitro* vs. *in vivo*, and the elimination of animal testing), the "greenness" of solvents, reagents, and waste materials, and the scientific robustness of the method(s) must be examined. Stability determination of a product is crucial, as it defines the shelf life of a biologically active component in a matrix, and becomes a sustainability consideration in terms of the plant volume required. Ideally, for a consistent product, bioactive constituent(s) should be assayed, independent of ubiquitous, interfering bioactive marker compounds [123, 124].

Another "greening" aspect is the use of biodegradable nano-constructs in cosmetics. These nano-devices (size-range of 1–100 nm) [125] have been in use in the cosmetic industry for about 30 years [126–128]. Nano-presentations promote the precise, durable delivery of chemicals to a target site and provide improved stability, thereby enhancing application consistency and sustainability. Examples include lipsticks, nail polishes, sunscreens, make-up, anti-ageing creams, and oral care products [129]. Nano-particles can maintain a sunscreen protection level with 50% less active ingredient [130], and nano-emulsions provide enhanced penetration of highly lipophilic compounds [131]. The conditions of use, with respect to toxicity, the variable chemistry of the nano-structures, and the human and environmental biodegradability, necessitate specific studies and sanction, prior to commercialization [132, 133].

9.2.4 Greening of Products: Degradation and Disposability

A long-standing concern for cosmetics with respect to a sustainable environment has been disposability and accumulation in the environment of residues and toxins [134]. A study of organic- and inorganic-chemicals of emerging concern (CECs) in cosmetics and hair care products identified ten compounds according to Annex XIII of the REACH Legislation [135]. Highest levels were for the presence of zinc oxide and titanium dioxide nano-particles in skin care products [136]. Although natural fragrances are highly desired [122], there are limitations to their use relating to volatility, lipophilicity, and susceptibility to oxidation [137]. Prolonging the stability of any natural product, including an essential oil, is therefore a sustainable activity, since the impact of heat, light, oxygen, etc. is reduced, and the desirable aroma maintained, producing an enhanced shelf life.

One innovation to address product degradation is delayed release based on micro-encapsulation, which captures and maintains the essential oil within a readily biodegradable material; examples include laundry adjuvants, body-washes, and shampoos [122, 138]; the various applied techniques have been reviewed [110, 139–142]. However, plastic micro-beads in cosmetics are now regarded as non-sustainable and a serious detrimental environmental issue [143]. Global efforts are underway to ban them from all face and body-wash products [144]. Chitin-based micro-beads, created from shrimp shell waste and polypropylene glycol, which can release 90% of the core ingredient within 7 h, may be more acceptable, sustainable, and environmentally acceptable [145]. Other scaffolds are also available [139, 146, 147].

Overall, consideration of sustainability of the ingredients from sourcing, the waste created during processing, and the disposal of the products and packaging, should be at the forefront of management policies and practices as a part of corporate social responsibility. These aspects are reviewed in the life cycle assessment (LCA) [148–151] of the ingredients in cosmetic products, which quantifies the environmental and energy performances, "the carbon footprint," of a product. It includes the cultivation, harvesting, transportation, processing of raw material, the packaging, and the transportation of the final product [152, 153]. Additionally, the consideration given to the use of all the materials and waste obtained from each process step, offers a more sustainable approach to the overall manufacturing process by reducing waste and justifying the mass of plant material harvested for cosmetics. The percentage difference of the input (fertilizers, pesticides, land space, water consumption, energy, etc.) and output ("waste" material) are a useful guide to develop frameworks for more sustainable practices. The use of "green indicators", including renewable carbon assessment, the E-factor, environmental risks, biodegradability, traceability, and biodiversity preservation, should be considered in the formulation and production of all ingredients in phytocosmetics.

A frequently used ingredient in cosmetic products is shea butter [154, 155]. The life cycle assessment of shea nut butter offers an interesting model for improving the sustainability of cosmetics and cosmeceutical ingredients (Figure 9.1). Typical for cosmetic ingredients, the supply costs of shea butter include labor, transportation, fuel, electric, and specifically for traditional shea nut butter, wood chips for burning, with the latter being mostly responsible for the percentage carbon footprint, addressed through using other heat sources for extraction [154]. However, although wood chip burning has a negative impact, the upcycling of the output (husks and kernel residue), may improve the overall "greening" of the supply chain. Both husks and kernel residue can

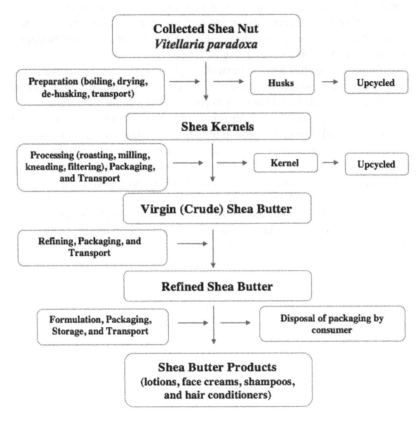

FIGURE 9.1   Life cycle assessment of shea butter, adapted from [154].

serve as sources of biomass [156] and activated carbon [157] and either be recycled in the supply chain, or serve as an alternative biofuel source in the areas of West Africa where shea nuts are processed [154, 155]. Other LCAs for cosmetic ingredients and packaging have been presented [158, 159].

9.3 GREEN CONSUMER

Consumer concern for contemporary environmental issues is reflected in the successful marketing of "green" products [160], which may involve lower solvent and power usage, reduced processing waste, environmentally friendly extraction protocols [161], and recyclable packaging, etc. [160, 162]. For cosmetics, it indicates a sustainable derivation from natural resources [163], an absence of synthetic chemicals for any purpose (active ingredient, fragrance, filler, colorant, diluent, preservative, etc.), and the disposability and biodegradation of the initial and final packaging [164].

Earlier studies had revealed that the highest interest in, and demand for, green cosmetic products was in the Asian-Pacific region [160, 165]. Recent surveys have revealed a willingness to pay (WTP) extra for a natural and sustainable cosmetic, recyclable packaging, and products not involving animal testing [165, 166]. The global growth of "The Body Shop" chain of stores since 1994 [167] prompted other corporations to examine their philosophies and practices regarding a more sustainable and reproducible cooperative approach to sourcing, and the elimination of animal-based toxicity testing [168, 169].

Another group of in-demand, natural cosmetic constituents are the essential oils (EOs), a mainstay ingredient in cosmetics and fragrances since 1600 BC. The botanical origins are diverse, and include plants in the families: Apiaceae, Asteraceae, Lamiaceae, Lauraceae, Myrtaceae, Pinaceae, Rutaceae, and Zingiberaceae [170], for the 2,000 plants of commercial value. Fragrances based on essential oils appear in a wide range of cosmetic products, either directly as perfumes, or indirectly in shampoos, bodywashes, and in various cleansers, creams, and ointments [122]. Consumers currently prefer these natural fragrances since they are less toxic, and being biodegradable, do not accrue in the biosphere [171], unlike the more slowly degrading synthetic fragrances [172]. In addition to fragrances, as a result of the anti-oxidant, anti-fungal, and anti-bacterial activities [173, 174], they are used in blends to enhance the stability of various products, which may reduce the use of synthetic preservatives in cosmetics [175].

Older, less "green", more energy-demanding processes for the recovery of essential oils, including steam distillation, solid-phase extraction, solvent extraction, and hydrodistillation [161], are being replaced by sustainable technologies, such as cold pressing, supercritical fluid (SFE), or microwave-assisted extraction (MAE), which do not involve hydrocarbon, chlorinated, or alcoholic solvents, and have reduced water and power requirements [176–179]. These innovations for the extraction of essential oils offer a more sustainable approach to their use as fragrances [122]. However, the life cycle assessment of citrus-based essential oils, such as orange, grapefruit, lime, and lemon, reveals a complicated view of their sustainability as fragrances. These oils are by-products of citrus farming, and the use of the peels and leaves for their essential oils enhances citrus farming sustainability, however, the input required (fertilizers, pesticides, fuel, energy, etc.) has a negative environmental impact [180]. There is a need for complementary and creative approaches using emerging technologies, to achieve sustainability and the further greening for phytocosmetics.

9.4 INTEGRATION OF EMERGING TECHNOLOGIES

Innovation in development, whether research or product-focused, is encapsulated within the new term "cyberecoethnopharmacolomics" [99], which represents the further integration of ecopharmacognosy [101, 102, 111] with many other disciplines and technologies, and provides a holistic approach to developing biologically active natural products. It conceptualizes the innovation opportunity of QSECA with sustainability and economics, aiming to improve processes and products on behalf of the patient, allow for adequate commercial development, and minimize the carbon footprint of the overall process. The morphemes are: "cyber" – the importance of diverse information systems before, during, and after conception and implementation, and includes automation; "eco" – the considerations of ecological impact of each stage in the process, and the sustainability of the utilized resource; "ethno" – the application of the background information derived from traditional medicine information; "pharmacol" – the determination of toxicity and biological activity for a health beneficent product; and "omics" – the taxonomics, the genomics, the extract metabolomics, and agronomics. Finally, there are all the economic aspects of the process of plant acquisition, processing, product creation, and delivery, possibly built on new business opportunities for societal benefit. For the successful transition of a plant to a marketable phytocosmetic product, integration of these factors in a sustainable manner is essential.

Many new technologies are available for integration to improve the existing, and the development of new, cosmetics and cosmeceuticals. Often, these technologies are the result of innovative sustainable developments which reduce or eliminate non-renewable resources. Some examples include: (i) the use of hand-held, remote sensing devices for in-field examination of the optimum time for harvesting an essential oil plant, (ii) the use of drones to seek and identify remote areas for plant collection, (iii) the routine use of high-field NMR- or HPLC/MS^n-based metabolomics to assess the status of an extract with respect to an established standard, (iv) the continuous re-assessment of analytical methods to eliminate adulterant plants or compounds, pesticides, and herbicides, (v) the development of rapid bioassays for a cosmeceutical bioassessment, and (vi) blockchain technologies. Integration of these strategies, and education regarding their importance, will help the patient make the healthy choice of a sustainable product, and enhance awareness on the greening and quality control in the cosmetic industry.

A recent consideration to enhance traceability, transparency, and trust throughout the supply chain and for the consumer is blockchain technology. This is a distributed ledgering system which allows for the construction of immutable transaction lists between parties, each of whom has access to the whole evolving chain [181]. Importantly, it allows for traceability from the field to the final product for all ingredients, including the packaging, and can provide evidence of sustainability and quality at each step in the manufacturing process towards the final product. Notably, it can provide reliable local economic benefits to the farming communities, transparency to all participants in the value chain, including the consumer, and enhance trustworthiness [182]. A large cosmetic company, in conjunction with a major supplier, has been experimenting with this technology for the production of vanilla from Madagascar [183], and the sensor-based tracing of wood, from sustainable harvest to the consumer purchase, has been described [184]. The technology has become a widely used standard in the food industry [185].

9.5 CONCLUSIONS

This brief chapter has highlighted some trends in sustainability for cosmetic and cosmeceutical products, particularly when a plant or an essential oil is incorporated. Issues related to establishing and maintaining the qualities from the field to the final product are emphasized with encouragement to operate with a life-cycle assessment of sustainable practices. From a buyers' perspective, considerable change is necessary. Regulatory issues supporting the consumer/patient are needed, including greater transparency in product labeling, particularly outside the European Union and Japan. More definitive considerations with respect to sustainability and environmental protection are required. Wider applications of green chemistry will represent cost savings long term and a marketing advantage. More research emphasis is essential to examine the biological effects of the cosmeceutical products, and to apply both chemical and biological assays for quality control. The promotion of plant surveys in the wild will assure maintenance of a sustainable supply chain as market opportunities expand if cultivation strategies are not being employed.

Long-term goals for cosmetics and cosmeceuticals production should focus on the transparency and traceability to enhance trust, integration of green technologies, the minimization of water usage and energy consumption, eliminating toxic solvents and environmentally degrading/accumulating excipients, expanded cultivation, improved biodegradable delivery systems, community investment strategies, and a purchaser-oriented balance of sustainability, social and environmental consciousness, and action is essential to require label transparency regarding the contents, their sourcing, the methods used to eliminate toxicity, and subsequently determine efficacy, together with the development of certification programs to support "green" processing practices, and a sustainable supply. In parallel, research is vital with respect to the future of plant sourcing and metabolite profiling in a time of climate change.

REFERENCES

1. United Nations Sustainable Development Goals. Available at: https://www.un.org/sustainabledevelopment/sustainable-development-goals/. 2015. Accessed on November 9, 2020.
2. Deming WE. Out of the Crisis. MIT Press, Cambridge, MA, USA, 2000, 507.
3. Newport C. Deep Work: Rules for Focused Success in a Distracted World. London: Piatkus Publishers; 2016:304.
4. Spangenberg JH, Pfahl S, Deller K. Towards indicators for institutional sustainability: lessons from an analysis of Agenda 21. Ecol Indic. 2002;2(1-2):61–77.
5. Elkington J. Enter the triple bottom line. In: Henriques A, Richardson J. eds. The Triple Bottom Line. London: Routledge; 2004. p. 1–16.
6. Liobikiené G, Bernatoniené J. Why determinants of green purchase cannot be treated equally? The case of green cosmetics: literature review. J Clean Prod. 2017;162:109–120.
7. Csorba L, Boglea V. Sustainable cosmetics: a major instrument in protecting the consumer's interest. Reg Bus Stud. 2011;3(Suppl 1):167–176.
8. Sahota A. Introduction to sustainability. In: Sahota A, ed. Sustainability: How the Cosmetics Industry is Greening Up. London: John Wiley & Sons; 2014. p. 1–16.

9. Nicholson PT. Ancient Egyptian Materials and Technology. Cambridge, UK: Cambridge University Press; 2000:175.
10. Chaudhri SK, Jain NK. History of cosmetics. Asian J Pharm. 2009;3(3): 164–167.
11. González-Minero FJ, Bravo-Díaz L. The use of plants in skin-care products, cosmetics and fragrances: past and present. Cosmetics. 2018;5(3):50.
12. Giorgio M, Trinei M, Migliaccio E, et al. Hydrogen peroxide: a metabolic by-product or a common mediator of ageing signals? Nature Rev Mol Cell Biol. 2007;8(9):722–728.
13. Callaghan TM, Wilhelm K-P. A review of ageing and an examination of clinical methods in the assessment of ageing skin. Part I: cellular and molecular perspectives of skin ageing. Int J Cosmetic Sci. 2008;30(5):313–322.
14. Kohl E, Steinbauer J, Landthaler M, et al. Skin ageing. J Eur Acad Dermatol Venereol. 2011;25(8):873–884.
15. Chermahini SH, Majid FAA, Sarmidi MR. Cosmeceutical value of herbal extracts as natural ingredients and novel technologies in anti-aging. J Med Plants Res. 2011;5(14):3074–3077.
16. Vaishali SK, Ashwini GC, Kshitija PD, Digambar NN. Cosmeceuticals an emerging concept: a comprehensive review. Int J Res Pharm Chem. 2013;3(2): 308–309.
17. Peng C, Wang X, Chen J, et al. Biology of ageing and role of dietary antioxidants. BioMed Res Int. 2014;831–841.
18. Vollmer DL, West WA, Lephart ED. Enhancing skin health: by oral administration of natural compounds and minerals with implications to the dermal microbiome. Int J Mol Sci. 2018;19(10):30–59.
19. Vermeer BJ, Gilchrest BA. Cosmeceuticals. A proposal for rational definition, evaluation, and regulation. Arch Dermatol. 1996;132(3):337–340.
20. Pieroni A, Quave CL, Villanelli ML, et al. Ethnopharmacognostic survey on the natural ingredients used in folk cosmetics, cosmeceuticals and remedies for healing skin diseases in the inland Marches, Central-Eastern Italy. J Ethnopharmacol. 2004;91(2-3):331–344.
21. Jenkins G. Molecular mechanisms of skin ageing. Mech Ageing Devel. 2002;123(7):801–810.
22. Steinbauer J, Landthaler M, et al. Skin ageing. J Eur Acad Dermatol Venereol. 2011;25(8):873–884.
23. Binic I, Lazarevic V, Ljubenovic M, et al. Skin ageing: natural weapons and strategies. Evid-Based Compl Alt Med. 2013;827248.
24. Krishnaiah D, Sarbatly R, Nithyanandam R. A review of the antioxidant potential of medicinal plant species. Food Bioprod Process. 2011;89(3):217–233.
25. Agati G, Azzarello E, Pollastri S, et al. Flavonoids as antioxidants in plants: location and functional significance. Plant Sci. 2012;196:67–76.
26. Sindhi V, Gupta V, Sharma K, et al. Potential applications of antioxidants - a review. J Pharm Res. 2013;7(9):828–835.
27. Liu D, Shi J, Ibarra AC, et al. The scavenging capacity and synergistic effects of lycopene, vitamin E, vitamin C, and β-carotene mixtures on the DPPH free radical. LWT-Food Sci Technol. 2008;41(7):1344–1349.
28. Foti MC, Amorati R. Non-phenolic radical-trapping antioxidants. J Pharm Pharmaol. 2009;61(11):1435–1448.

29. Baschieri A, Ajvazi MD, Tonfack JLF, et al. Explaining the antioxidant activity of some common non-phenolic components of essential oils. Food Chem. 2017;232:656–663.
30. Gordon MH. Dietary antioxidants in disease prevention. Nat Prod Rep. 1996;13(4):265–273.
31. Zhang Y-J, Gan R-Y, Li S, et al. Antioxidant phytochemicals for the prevention and treatment of chronic diseases. Molecules 2015;20(12):21138–21156.
32. Serri R, Iorizzo M. Cosmeceuticals: focus on topical retinoids in photoaging. Clin Dermatol. 2008;26(6):633–635.
33. Sofen B, Prado G, Emer J. Melasma and post inflammatory hyperpigmentation: management update and expert opinion. Skin Ther Lett. 2016;21(1):1–7.
34. Lee HE, Ko JY, Kim YH, et al. A double-blind randomized controlled comparison of APDDR-0901, a novel cosmeceutical formulation, and 0.1% adapalene gel in the treatment of mild-to-moderate acne vulgaris. Eur J Dermatol. 2011;21(6):959–965.
35. Barros BS, Zaenglein AL. The use of cosmeceuticals in acne: help or hoax? Am J Clin Dermatol. 2017;18(2):159–163.
36. Vogelgesang B, Abdul-Malak N, Reymermier C, et al. On the effects of a plant extract of *Orthosiphon stamineus* on sebum-related skin imperfections. Intl J Cosmetic Sci. 2011;33(1):44–52.
37. Endly DC, Miller RA. Oily skin: a review of treatment options. J Clin Aesthet Dermatol. 2017;10(8):49–55.
38. Wuthi-Udomlert M, Chotipatoomwan P, Panyadee S, et al. 2011. Inhibitory effect of formulated lemongrass shampoo on *Malassezia furfur*: a yeast associated with dandruff. SE Asian J Trop Med Pub Health. 2011;42(2):363–369.
39. Emer J, Waldorf H, Berson D. Botanicals and anti-inflammatories: natural ingredients for rosacea. Semin Cutan Med Surg. 2011;30:148–155.
40. Draelos ZD. Cosmeceuticals for rosacea. Clin Dermatol. 2017;35(2):213–217.
41. Gubitosa J, Rizzi V, Fini P, et al. Hair care cosmetics: from traditional shampoo to solid clay and herbal shampoo, a review. Cosmetics. 2019;6(1):13.
42. Rathi V, Rathi J, Tamizharasi S, et al. Plants used for hair growth promotion: a review. Pharmacogn Rev. 2008;2(3):185.
43. D'Amelio, FS. Botanicals - A Phytocosmetic Desk Reference. Boca Raton: CRC Press; 1999:361.
44. Talal A, Feda NM. Plants used in cosmetics. Phytother Res. 2003;17(9):987–1000.
45. Thornfeldt C. Cosmeceuticals containing herbs: fact, fiction, and future. Dermatol Surg. 2005;31(s1):873–881.
46. Berger RG, ed. Flavours and Fragrances: Chemistry, Bioprocessing and Sustainability. Berlin: Springer Science & Business Media; 2007:648.
47. Sahota A, ed. Sustainability: How the Cosmetics Industry is Greening Up. Chichester: John Wiley & Sons Ltd.; 2014:363.
48. Gurib-Fakim A, ed. Novel Plant Bioresources: Applications in Food, Medicine and Cosmetics. Chichester: John Wiley & Sons Ltd.; 2014:512.
49. Fonseca-Santos B, Corrêa MA, Chorilli M. Sustainability, natural and organic cosmetics: consumer, products, efficacy, toxicological and regulatory considerations. Braz J Pharm Sci. 2015;51(1):17–26.
50. Joshi LS, Pawar HA. Herbal cosmetics and cosmeceuticals: an overview. Nat Prod Chem Res. 2015;3(2):170.

51. Anonymous. State of the World's Plants 2017. Royal Botanic Gardens Kew. 2017:100. Available at: https://stateoftheworldsplants.org/. Accessed on October 18, 2020.

52. Cordell GA. The Convention on Biological Diversity and its impact on natural product research. In: Buss AD, Butler MS, eds. Natural product chemistry for drug discovery. Cambridge: Royal Society of Chemistry Publishing; 2010. p. 81–139.

53. Chen S, Pang V, Song J et al. A renaissance in herbal medicine identification: from morphology to DNA. Biotechnol Adv. 2014;32(7):1237–1244.

54. Mak CY, Mok CS. Molecular identification of *Lodoicea maldivica* (coco de mer) seeds. Chin Med. 2011;6:34.

55. Fong HHS, Simon JE, Regalado J. WHO Guidelines on Good Agricultural and Collection Practices (GACP) for Medicinal Plants. Geneva: World Health Organization; 2003:80.

56. Leaman DJ. Sustainable wild collection of medicinal and aromatic plants: development of an international standard. In: Bogers RJ, Craker LE, Lange D, eds. Medicinal and Aromatic Plants, Volume 18; Berlin: Springer; 2006. 97–107.

57. Medicinal Plant Specialist Group. International Standard for Sustainable Wild Collection of Medicinal and Aromatic Plants (ISSC-MAP). Version 1.0. Bonn; Bundesamt für Naturschutz (BfN), MPSG/SSC/IUCN, WWF Germany, and TRAFFIC, BfN Skripten 195; 2007:38.

58. Schippmann UWE, Leaman D, Cunningham AB. A comparison of cultivation and wild collection of medicinal and aromatic plants under sustainability aspects. In: Bogers RJ, Craker LE, Lange D, eds. Medicinal and Aromatic Plants, Volume 18. Berlin: Springer; 2006. 75–95.

59. Alam AF, Er AC, Begum H. Malaysian oil palm industry: prospect and problem. J Food Agric Environ. 2015;13(2):143–148.

60. Paterson RRM, Lima N. Climate change affecting oil palm agronomy, and oil palm cultivation increasing climate change, require amelioration. Ecol Evol. 2018;8(1):452–461.

61. Schippmann U, Leaman DJ, Cunningham AB. Impact of cultivation and gathering of medicinal plants on biodiversity: global trends and issues. Biodiversity and the Ecosystem Approach in Agriculture, Forestry and Fisheries. Ninth Regular Session of the Commission on Genetic Resources for Food and Agriculture. Rome, 12–13 October 2002. Inter-Departmental Working Group on Biological Diversity for Food and Agriculture. FAO, Rome. 2002:21.

62. Schmidt BM. Responsible use of medicinal plants for cosmetics. HortScience. 2012;47(8):985–991.

63. Hamilton AC. Medicinal plants, conservation and livelihoods. Biodivers Conserv. 2004;13(8):1477–1517.

64. Choudhary D, Pandit BH, Kala SP, et al. Upgrading bay leaf farmers in value chains - strategies for improving livelihoods and poverty reduction from Udayapur district of Nepal. Soc Nat Resour. 2014;27(10):1057–1073.

65. Choudhary D, Kala SP, Todaria NP, et al. Upgrading mountain people in medicinal and aromatic plants value chains: lessons for sustainable management and income generation from Uttarakhand, India. Int J Sustain Devel World Ecol. 2013;20(1):45–53.

66. Chandra P, Sharma V. Strategic marketing prospects for developing sustainable medicinal and aromatic plants businesses in the Indian Himalayan region. Small-scale For. 2018;17(4):423–441.
67. Akerele O, Heywood V, Synge H, eds. Conservation of Medicinal Plants. Cambridge: Cambridge University Press; 1991: 382.
68. Shinwari ZK. Medicinal plants research in Pakistan. J Med Plants Res. 2010;4(3):161–176.
69. Magoro MD, Masoga MA, Mearns MA. Traditional health practitioners' practices and the sustainability of extinction-prone traditional medicinal plants. Int J Afr Renaiss Stud. 2010;5(2):229–241.
70. Louhaichi M, Salkini AK, Estita HE, et al. Initial assessment of medicinal plants across the Libyan Mediterranean coast. Adv Environ Biol. 2011;5(2): 359–370.
71. Amujoyegbe BJ, Agbedahunsi JM, Amujoyegbe OO. Cultivation of medicinal plants in developing nations: means of conservation and poverty alleviation. Int J Med Arom Plants. 2012;2(2):345–353.
72. Williams VL, Victor JE, Crouch NR. Red listed medicinal plants of South Africa: status, trends, and assessment challenges. S Afr J Bot. 2013;86:23–35.
73. Sharma S, Thokchom R. A review on endangered medicinal plants of India and their conservation. J Crop Weed. 2014;10(2):205–218.
74. Seidler-Łożykowska K, Mordalski R, Kucharski W, et al. Yielding and quality of lavender flowers (*Lavandula angustifolia* Mill.) from organic cultivation. Acta Sci Pol, Hort Cultus. 2014;13(6):173–183.
75. Stanev S, Zagorcheva T, Atanassov I. Lavender cultivation in Bulgaria – 21st century developments, breeding challenges and opportunities. Bulg J Agric Sci. 2016;22(4):584–590.
76. Giannoulis KD, Evangelopoulos V, Gougoulias N, et al. Could bio-stimulators affect flower, essential oil yield, and its composition in organic lavender (*Lavandula angustifolia*) cultivation? Ind Crop Prod. 2010;154:112611.
77. Cordell GA, Colvard MD. Natural products and traditional medicine – turning on a paradigm. J Nat Prod. 2012;75(3):514–525.
78. Cordell GA. Ecopharmacognosy – the responsibilities of natural product research to sustainability. Phytochem Lett. 2015;11:332–346.
79. Cordell GA. Ecopharmacognosy and the globalization of traditional medicine. Ind J Tradit Knowl. 2015;14(4):595–604.
80. Thorpe TA. History of plant tissue culture. Mol Biotechnol. 2007;37(2): 169–180.
81. Barbulova A, Apone F, Colucci G. Plant cell cultures as source of cosmetic active ingredients. Cosmetics. 2014;1(2):94–104.
82. Eibl R, Meier P, Stutz I, et al. Plant cell culture technology in the cosmetics and food industries: current state and future trends. Appl Microbiol Biotechnol. 2018;102(20):8661–8675.
83. Suvanto J, Nohynek L, Seppänen-Laakso T, et al. Variability in the production of tannins and other polyphenols in cell cultures of 12 Nordic plant species. Planta. 2017;246:227–241.
84. Trehan S, Michniak-Kohn B, Beri K. Plant stem cells in cosmetics: current trends and future directions. Future Sci OA. 2017;3(4):FSO226.
85. Di Martino O, Tito A, de Lucia A, et al. *Hibiscus syriacus* extract from an established cell culture stimulates skin wound healing. Biomed Res Int. 2017;7932019.

86. Dal Toso R, Melandri F. Sustainable sourcing of natural food ingredients by plant cell cultures. Agro Food Ind Hi Tech. 2011;22:30–32.
87. Dal Toso R, Melandri F. *Echinacea angustifolia* cell culture extract. Nutrafoods. 2011;10(4):19–25.
88. Belser E. Anti-ageing hair care: preventing hair loss and ensuring fuller hair. COSSMA. 2015;1:10–11.
89. Schürch C, Blum P, Zülli F. Potential of plant cells in culture for cosmetic application. Phytochem Rev. 2008;7:599–605.
90. Schmid D, Zülli F. Use of plant cell cultures for a sustainable production of innovative ingredients. SOFW J. 2012;138(9):2–10.
91. Morus M, Baran M, Rost-Rozkowska M, et al. Plant stem cells as innovation in cosmetics. Acta Pol Pharm. 2014;71(5):701–707.
92. Zappelli C, Barbulova A, Apone F, et al. Effective active ingredients obtained through biotechnology. Cosmetics. 2016;3(4):39.
93. Teimoori-Boghsani Y, Ganjeali A, Cernava T, et al. Endophytic fungi of native *Salvia abrotanoides* plants reveal high taxonomic diversity and unique profiles of secondary metabolites. Front Microbiol. 2010;10:3013.
94. Zhang Y, Li F, Huang F, et al. Metabolomics analysis reveals variation in *Schisandra chinensis* metabolites from different origins. J Sep Sci. 2014;37(6):731–737.
95. Lee J, Jung Y, Shin J-H, et al. Secondary metabolite profiling of *Curcuma* species grown at different locations using GC/TOF and UPLC/Q-TOF MS. Molecules. 2014;19(7):9535–9551.
96. Zhao, Y, Zhao J, Zhao C, et al. A metabolomics study delineating geographical location-associated primary metabolic changes in the leaves of growing tobacco plants by GC-MS and CE-MS. Sci Rep. 2015;5:16346.
97. Mishra T. Climate change and production of secondary metabolites in medicinal plants: a review. Int J Herb Med. 2016;4(4):27–30.
98. Anonymous. Cosmetics Labeling Claims. Available at: https://www.fda.gov/cosmetics/cosmetics-labeling-claims/cosmeceutical. Accessed on October 18, 2020.
99. Cordell GA. Cyberecoethnopharmacolomics. J Ethnopharmacol. 2019;244:112–134.
100. Cordell GA. Cognate and cognitive ecopharmacognosy – in an anthropogenic era. Phytochem Lett. 2017;20:540–549.
101. Cordell GA. Sixty challenges – a 2030 perspective on natural products and medicines security. Nat Prod Commun. 2017;12(8):1371–1379.
102. Cordell GA. Alice, benzene, and coffee: the ABC's of ecopharmacognosy. Nat Prod Commun. 2015;10(12):2195–2202.
103. Morris CA, Avorn J. Internet marketing of herbal products. J Am Med Assoc. 2003;290(11):1505–1509.
104. Tsai TC, Hantasch BM. Cosmeceutical agents: a comprehensive review of the literature. Clin Med Insights Dermatol. 2008;1(1):1–20.
105. Faber S. Environmental Working Group. On cosmetic safety US trails more than 40 nations. 2019. https://www.ewg.org/news-and-analysis/2019/03/cosmetics-safety-us-trails-more-40-nations.
106. Dorato S. General concepts: current legislation on cosmetics in various countries. In: Salvador A, Chisvert A, eds. Analysis of Cosmetic Products. Amsterdam: Elsevier; 2018. 3–37.

107. European Parliament & Council of the European Union. Regulation (EC) No 1223/2009 of the European Parliament and of the Council on Cosmetic Products. Off J Eur Union. 2009, L 342/59–L 342/209. Available at: https://ec.europa. eu/health/sites/health/files/endocrine_disruptors/docs/cosmetic_1223_2009_regulation_en.pdf. Accessed on October 18, 2020.

108. United States Food and Drug Administration. Is it a cosmetic, a drug, or both? (Or is it soap?) (2012). Available at: http://www.fda.gov/Cosmetics/GuidanceRegulation/LawsRegulations/ucm074201.htm#Intended_use. Accessed on October 18, 2020.

109. Franca CCV, Ueno HM. Green cosmetics: perspectives and challenges in the context of green chemistry. Desenvolv Meio Ambient. 2020;53:133–150.

110. Carvalho IT, Estevinho BN, Santos L. Application of microencapsulated essential oils in cosmetic and personal healthcare products – a review. Int J Cosmetic Sci. 2016;38(2):109–119.

111. Cordell GA., Ecopharmacognosy – why natural products matter – now and for the future. Thai Bull Pharm Sci. 2013;13(1):1–9.

112. McNeill JR. Something New Under the Sun: An Environmental History of the Twentieth-Century World. New York: W.W. Norton & Company, Inc.; 2000:421.

113. Anastas P, Warner J. Green Chemistry: Theory and Practice. New York; Oxford University Press, Inc.; 2000:135.

114. Anastas PT, Zimmerman JB. Design through the 12 principles of green engineering. Environ Sci Technol. 2003;37(5):94A–101A.

115. Shah AA, Hasan F, Hameed A, et al. Biological degradation of plastics: a comprehensive review. Biotechnol Adv. 2008;26(3):246–265.

116. Beerling, J. Green formulations and ingredients. In: Sahota A, ed. Sustainability: How the Cosmetics Industry is Greening Up. London: John Wiley & Sons; 2014: 197–216.

117. Pereira de Carvalho A, Barbieri JC. Innovation and sustainability in the supply chain of a cosmetics company: a case study. J Technol Manage Innov. 2012;7(2):144–156.

118. Kim H, Verpoorte R. Sample preparation for plant metabolomics. Phytochem Anal. 2010;21(1):4–13.

119. Schripsema J. Application of NMR in plant metabolomics: techniques, problems and prospects. Phytochem Anal. 2010;21(1):14–21.

120. Ernst M, Silva DB, Silva RR, et al. Mass spectrometry in plant metabolomics strategies: from analytical platforms to data acquisition and processing. Nat Prod Rep. 2014;31(6):784–806.

121. Women's Voices for the Earth. Unpacking the fragrance industry: policy failures, the trade secret myth and public health. Missoula; Women's Voices for the Earth; 2018:16.

122. Delisi R, Pagliaro M, Ciriminna R. Sustainability. Green fragrances: a critically important technology for the new cosmetic industry. Hsehld Pers Care Today. 2016;11(5):67–71.

123. Baell JB. Feeling nature's PAINS: natural products, natural product drugs, and pan assay interference compounds (PAINS). J Nat Prod. 2016;79(3):616–628.

124. Bisson J, McAlpine B, Friesen JB, et al. Can invalid bioactives undermine natural product-based drug discovery? J Med Chem. 2016;59(5):1671–1690.

125. Regulation (EC) No 1223/2009 of the European Parliament and of the Council of 30 November 2009 on Cosmetic Products (recast). Off J Eur Union L342/59-209.

126. Pastrana H, Avila A, Tsai CSJ. Nanomaterials in cosmetic products: the challenges with regard to current legal frameworks and consumer exposure. NanoEthics. 2018;12:123–137.
127. Carrouel F, Viennot S, Ottolenghi L, et al. Nanoparticles as anti-microbial, anti-inflammatory, and remineralizing agents in oral care cosmetics: a review of the current situation. Nanomaterials. 2020;10(1):140.
128. Revia RA, Wagner BA, Zhang M. A portable electrospinner for nanofiber synthesis and its application for cosmetic treatment of alopecia. Nanomaterials. 2019;9(9):1317.
129. Fytianos G, Rahdar A, Kyzas GZ. Nanomaterials in cosmetics: recent updates. Nanomaterials. 2020;10(5):979.
130. Wissing SA, Müller RH. Cosmetic applications for solid lipid nanoparticles (SLN). Int J Pharm. 2003;254(1):65–68.
131. Zülli F, Belser E, Schmid D, et al. Preparation and properties of coenzyme Q10 nanoemulsions. Cosmet Sci Technol. 2006;40–46.
132. Singh P, Nanda A. Nanotechnology in cosmetics: a boon or bane? Toxicol Environ Chem. 2012;94(8):1467–1479.
133. Antignac E, Nohynek GJ, Re T, et al. Safety of botanical ingredients in personal care products/cosmetics. Food Chem Toxicol. 2011;49(2):324–341.
134. REACH Online. Annex XIII: criteria for the identification of persistent, bioaccumulative and toxic substances, and very persistent and very bioaccumulative substances. Available at: https://reachonline.eu/reach/en/annex-xiii.html. Accessed on November 15, 2020.
135. Prothero A, McDonagh P. Producing environmentally acceptable cosmetics? The impact of environmentalism on the United Kingdom cosmetics and toiletries industry. J Market Manage. 1992;8(2):147–166.
136. Dhanirama D, Gronow J, Voulvoulis N. Cosmetics as a potential source of environmental contamination in the UK. Environ Technol. 2012;33(14):1597–1608.
137. Turek C, Stintzing FC. Stability of essential oils: a review. Comp Rev Food Sci Food Safe. 2013;12(1):40–53.
138. Ciriminna R, Pagliaro M. Sol-gel microencapsulation of odorants and flavors: opening the route to sustainable fragrances and aromas. Chem Soc Rev. 2013;42(24):9243–9250.
139. Chanchal D, Swarnlata S. Novel approaches in herbal cosmetics. J Cosmet Dermatol. 2008;7(2):89–95.
140. Ammala A. Biodegradable polymers as encapsulation materials for cosmetics and personal care markets. Int J Cosmetic Sci. 2013;35(2):113–124.
141. Martins IM, Barreiro MF, Coelho M, et al. Microencapsulation of essential oils with biodegradable polymeric carriers for cosmetic applications. Chem Eng J. 2014;245:191–200.
142. Nam HC, Park WH. Aliphatic polyester-based biodegradable microbeads for sustainable cosmetics. ACS Biomater Sci Eng. 2020;6(4):2440–2449.
143. Rochman CM., Kross SM, Armstrong JB, et al. Scientific evidence supports a ban on microbeads. Environ Sci Technol. 2015;49(18):10759–10761.
144. Guerranti C, Martellini T, Perra G, et al. Microplastics in cosmetics: environmental issues and needs for global bans. Environ Toxicol Pharmacol. 2019;68:75–79.

145. King CA, Shamshina JL, Zavgorodnya O, et al. Porous chitin microbeads for more sustainable cosmetics. ACS Sustain Chem Eng. 2017;5(12):11660–11667.
146. Bombardelli E, Cum SB, Loggia R, et al. Complexes between phospholipids and vegetal derivatives of biological interest. Fitoterapia. 1989;60:1–9.
147. Bombardelli E, Cristoni A, Morazzoni P. Phytosomes in functional cosmetics. Fitoterapia. 1994;65(5):387–389.
148. Finnveden G, Hauschild MZ, Ekvall T, et al. Recent developments in life cycle assessment. J Environ Manage. 2009;91(1):1–21.
149. Guinée JB, Heijungs R, Huppes G, et al. Life cycle assessment: past, present, and future. Environ Sci Technol. 2011;45(1):90–96.
150. Guinée J. Handbook on life cycle assessment operational guide to the ISO standards. Int J Life Cycle Assess. 2002;7(5):311–313.
151. Dewulf J, Benini L, Mancini L,. Rethinking the area of protection "natural resources" in life cycle assessment. Environ Sci Technol. 2015;49(9):5310–5317.
152. Bom S, Jorge J, Ribeiro HM, et al. A step forward on sustainability in the cosmetics industry: a review. J Clean Prod. 2019;225:270–290.
153. Civancik-Uslu D, Puig R, Voigt S, et al. Improving the production chain with LCA and eco-design: application to cosmetic packaging. Resour Conserv Recy. 2019;151:104475.
154. Glew D, Lovett PN. Life cycle analysis of shea butter use in cosmetics: from parklands to product, low carbon opportunities. J Clean Prod. 2014;68:73–80.
155. Naughton CC, Zhang Q, Mihelcic JR. Modelling energy and environmental impacts of traditional and improved shea butter production in West Africa for food security. Sci Total Environ. 2017;576:284–291.
156. Oviasogie PO, Odewale JO, Aisueni NO, et al. Production, utilization and acceptability of organic fertilizers using palms and shea tree as sources of biomass. Afr J Agric Res. 2013;8(27):3483–3494.
157. Amola LA, Kamgaing T, Tchuifon DR, et al. Activated carbons based on shea nut shells (*Vitellaria paradoxa*): optimization of preparation by chemical means using response surface methodology and physicochemical characterization. J Mater Sci Chem Eng. 2020;8(8):53–72.
158. Pérez-López P, González-García S, Jeffryes C, et al. Life cycle assessment of the production of the red antioxidant carotenoid astaxanthin by microalgae: from lab to pilot scale. J Clean Prod. 2014;64:332–344.
159. Secchi M, Castellani V, Collina E, et al. Assessing eco-innovations in green chemistry: Life Cycle Assessment (LCA) of a cosmetic product with a bio-based ingredient. J Clean Prod. 2016;129:269–281.
160. Chin J, Jiang BC, Mufidah I, et al. The investigation of consumers' behavior intention in using green skincare products: a pro-environmental behavior model approach. Sustainability 2018;10(11):3922.
161. Azmir J, Zaidul ISM, Rahman MM, et al. Techniques for extraction of bioactive compounds from plant materials: a review. J Food Eng. 2013;117(4):426–436.
162. Zappelli C, Barbulova A, Apone F, Colucci G, et al. Effective active ingredients obtained through biotechnology. Cosmetics. 2016;3(4):39.
163. Lin Y, Yang S, Hanifah H, Iqbal Q. An exploratory study of consumer attitudes toward green cosmetics in the UK market. Adm Sci. 2018;8(4):71.

164. Campion J-F, Barre R, Gilbert L. Innovating to reduce the environmental footprint, the L'Oréal example. In: Sahota A, ed. Sustainability: How the Cosmetics Industry is Greening Up. London: John Wiley & Sons; 2014: 31–46.
165. Amberg N, Fogarassy C. Green consumer behavior in the cosmetics market. Resources. 2019;8(3):137.
166. Joung SH, Park SW, Ko YJ. Willingness to pay for eco-friendly products: case of cosmetics. Asia Market J. 2014;15(4):33–49.
167. Philippe M, Didillon B, Gilbert L. Industrial commitment to green and sustainable chemistry: using renewable materials & developing eco-friendly processes and ingredients in cosmetics. Green Chem. 2012;14(4):952–956.
168. Utroske D. Sustainably sourced sandalwood oil coming to the fragrance industry. https://www.cosmeticsdesign.com/Article/2015/04/01/Sustainably-sourced-sandalwood-oil-coming-to-the-fragrance-industry. Accessed on October 18, 2020.
169. Sielaff S, Witter C, Tenge C. Symrise and vanilla: tradition, strategy, and total commitment. In: D'heur M, ed. Sustainable value chain management. Berlin: Springer; 2014: 185–205.
170. Heinrich M, Williamson EM, Gibbons S, et al. Fundamentals of Pharmacognosy and Phytotherapy, 3rd Ed. Amsterdam: Elsevier Health Sciences, 2017:360.
171. Regnault-Roger C, Vincent C, Arnason JT, Essential oils in insect control: low-risk products in a high-stakes world. Annu Rev Entomol. 2012;57:405–424.
172. Peck AM, Linebaugh EK, Hornbuckle KC. Synthetic musk fragrances in Lake Erie and Lake Ontario sediment cores. Environ Sci Technol. 2006;40(18):5629–5635.
173. Bakkali F, Averbeck S, Averbeck D, et al. Biological effects of essential oils - a review. Food Chem Toxicol. 2008;46(2):446–475.
174. Shaaban HAE, El-Ghorab AH, Shibamoto T. Bioactivity of essential oils and their volatile aroma components: review. J Essent Oil Res. 2012;24(2):203–212.
175. Ku J-E, Han H-S, Song J-H. The recent trend of the natural preservative used in cosmetics. Kor J Aesthet Cosmetol. 2013;11(5):835–844.
176. Lucchesi ME, Chemat F, Smadja J. Solvent-free microwave extraction of essential oil from aromatic herbs: comparison with conventional hydro-distillation. J Chromatogr A. 2004;1043(2):323–327.
177. Pereira CG, Prado JM, Angela M, et al. Economic evaluation of natural product extraction processes. In: Rostagno MA, Prado JM, eds. Natural Product Extraction: Principles and Applications. Cambridge: RSC Publishing; 2013: 516.
178. Capuzzo A, Maffei ME, Occhipinti A. Supercritical fluid extraction of plant flavors and fragrances. Molecules. 2013;18(6):7194–7238.
179. Ciriminna R, Carnaroglio D, Delisi R, et al. Industrial feasibility of natural products extraction with microwave technology. Chem Select. 2016;1(3):549–555.
180. Beccali M, Cellura M, Iudicello M, et al. Life cycle assessment of Italian citrus-based products. Sensitivity analysis and improvement scenarios. J Environ Manage. 2010;91(7):1415–1428.
181. Kouhizadeh M, Sarkis J. Blockchain practices, potentials, and perspectives in greening supply chains. Sustainability. 2018;10(10):3652.
182. Heinrich, M, Scotti F, Booker A, et al. Unblocking high-value botanical value chains: is there a role for blockchain systems? Front Pharmacol. 2019;10:396.

183. Webwire. ELC and Aveda pilot blockchain tech in Madagascan vanilla supply chain. Available at: https://www.webwire.com/ViewPressRel_print. asp?aId=265591. Accessed on November 13, 2020.
184. Figorilli S, Antonucci F, Costa C, et al. A blockchain implementation prototype for the electronic open source traceability of wood along the whole supply chain. Sensors. 2018;18:E3133.
185. Behnke K, Janssen MFWHA. Boundary conditions for traceability in food supply chains using blockchain technology. Int J Inf Manage. 2020;52:101969.

Index

Note: Locators in *italics* indicate figures and in **bold** indicate tables in the text.